ESSENTIAL OILS AND ME

Kathleen Pepper

Illustrated by Bodel Rikys

'Let fragrance guide you'

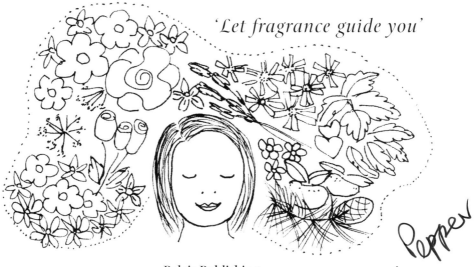

Polair Publishing
P O BOX 34886 · LONDON W8 6YR
www.polairpublishing.co.uk

Kathleen Pepper

First published April 2007

© Kathleen Pepper, 2007
Drawings © Bodel Rikys, 2007

British Library Cataloguing-in-Publication Data
A catalogue record for this book is available from the British Library

ISBN 978-1-905398-12-6

Dedication
I would like to dedicate this book to Ylana Hayward, who was my teacher of meditation
in 1975. It was on her ninetieth birthday that I finished this book.

Acknowledgments
I cannot adequately thank my husband, Roy, for his patience in helping me with the computer. I
should like to acknowledge my gratitude to Gabriel Mojay, Principal of The Institute of Traditional
Herbal Medicine and Aromatherapy, with whom I studied in 1995. He gave me deeper insights into the
qualities of essential oils, including their energetic (vibrational) properties, and many of the keynotes
used for the essential oils discussed in this work. For the brief historical overview of the use of plant
materials, THE AROMATHERAPY WORKBOOK, by Shirley Price (Thorsons, 1993) has been invaluable. Thanks
are also due to Colum Hayward for his helpful support and advice.

Set in Arepo at the Publishers
and printed in Great Britain by Cambridge University Press

CONTENTS

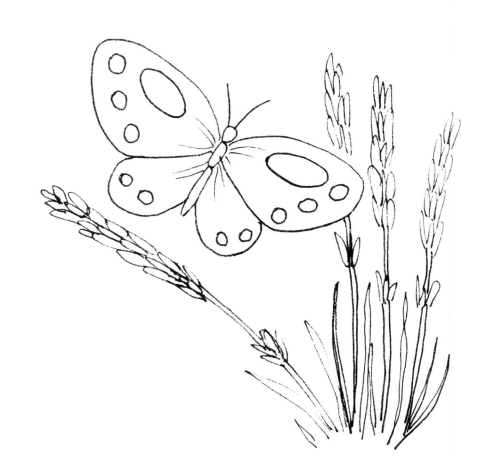

1. USING ESSENTIAL OILS AND PLANT MATERIALS IN MEDITATION

Love is the only thing that opens our hearts. Essential oils carry the love vibration of flowers and healing herbs
(Paracelsus)

Introduction

THE IDEA for this little book arose from more than thirty years' experience of using essential oils as an aid to meditation and in my work as a clinical aromatherapist. For most of this time I have been teaching and facilitating workshops in several therapeutic areas, especially yoga, relaxation and meditation, massage and aromatherapy, and 'Connecting with Angels'. I usually use essential oils in a diffuser or vaporizer to enhance the atmosphere in the room. Essential oils vaporize cleanly and release their aroma without smoke or ash. People often ask me to supply the particular blend of oils used. This is easier said than done, since I usually make a unique blend for the purpose of the event, so it can be different each time. In 2006, I was asked to give a talk at the Summer Festival of the White Eagle Lodge in Hampshire. It was about the history of essential oils and plant materials to enhance the benefits of meditation. I also sold a meditation oil blend I had formulated, which proved popular. The audience asked where they could find out more information and suggested I write a book about the topic, so here it is. While writing this book, I used an electric essential oil vaporizer to evaporate the particular oil I was describing. The meditations given here were directly inspired by this use of the oils. Others are culled from my meditation diaries, which I have kept over a period of more than thirty years. These meditations can be used as a starting point, but always follow your own inspiration.

We shall not be discussing fully the therapeutic and healing properties of the essential oils, as many books already do this.

From the time of ancient Egypt to the present,

plants and herbs have traditionally been used to induce a meditative state. It is believed that certain essential oils can be used to lead the mind from the every day state into one of relaxation and meditation. Modern scientists use a piece of equipment called an electroencephalograph to measure the rate of brain waves. In meditation, the rate of the brain waves alters. To quote from a scientific report in another book in this series, 'Evidence that meditation leads to an increase in alpha waves is extensive.... A characteristic brain-wave pattern of long-term meditators includes strong bursts of frontally dominant theta rhythms, during which meditators report peaceful, drifting, and generally pleasant experiences with intact self-awareness.*

There are several ways of using essential oils as an aid to meditation. They can be evaporated over water using a tea light or in an electric diffuser or vaporizer. They can be used directly on the body, —for example, on the chest over the heart chakra or the third eye (eyebrow centre), on the inside of the wrists or inner anklebones where the pulses are. If used directly on the skin, essential oils should be diluted first in some vegetable oil, like almond or jojoba, as

*From WHY MEDITATION WORKS by James Baltzell, MD (Polair Guides, 2006).

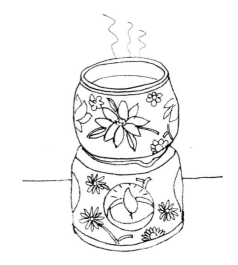

they are very powerful and can irritate the skin when used neat. In all cases, use only a safe amount of two or three drops.

We find that it was only in the twentieth century that oils were extracted and used for their aroma, hence the coining of the word 'aromatherapy'. Historically, the whole plant was used, as in herbalism. The word aromatherapy has recently come to be used in cosmetics and pharmaceuticals as a selling attraction. However, the earliest evidence for using plants is found in cave paintings in the Dordogne region of France, dating from about eighteen thousand years ago. These paintings are thought to show how plants were generally used for medicinal purposes.

There are many ways to obtain aromatic extracts from plants. These include expression of the peel, as with citrus fruits; enfleurage, where jasmine flowers are laid on trays of fat or oil to extract the perfume; maceration and solvent extraction, as well as the usual method of distillation. Distillation was traditionally used to extract exotic flower waters and essences for use in perfumes, such as rose. The amount of essential oils present in the petals is very small. You need sixty thousand roses to make 28 grams (a fluid ounce) of rose essential oil. That is, twenty-five roses produce one drop of oil, making rose oil very expensive. If, as a child, you tried to make rose perfume by soaking rose petals, this is the reason that the result was disappointing, to say the least!

The earliest evidence for extracting aromatic substances from plants is found in Egypt and India, about five thousand years ago. In both countries, the use of plants played an important role, linking religion and medicine together. In India, there has been continuous use of plants in Ayurvedic medicine until the present. One of the oldest references to using plants is found in the Vedas. In Mohenjo Dara, an ancient city excavated in the Indus Valley in what is now Pakistan, there is archaeological evidence of a method of primitive distillation. Plant material, such as sandalwood, ginger, myrrh, cinnamon and coriander, was placed in a clay vessel, then covered with a thick layer of sheep's fleece and heated. The fleece would gradually be saturated with the essential oil from condensed steam and, when cool, it could be squeezed to produce the oil. It is thought a similar system was also used in Egypt.

There is plenty of information about the use of plants in Egypt and the Nile is known as the cradle of medicine. Cedarwood, frankincense, myrrh and cinnamon were in common use. As well as the primitive means of distillation noted, the Egyptians used fats or waxes to extract fat- or wax-soluble molecules from plants, and paintings of jars containing such substances are seen in Egyptian tombs. The Egyptians were so successful in their use and knowledge of plants that embalmed bodies are still preserved three thousand years later. Perfumery was associated with the Egyptian priesthood, who worked out the formulas that were used by the pharaohs to anoint themselves for ceremony, war and love. Special incense called kyphi was burnt in offering at sunset to

Ra, the Egyptian sun god. There are several recipes for kyphi and it included such ingredients as wine, honey, raisins, myrrh, cardomom, juniper, mint, cypress, spikenard, cassia and cinnamon. It was reputed to heal the soul. The Egyptians were not the only people who used aromas or resins in religious ceremonies. Assyrians, Babylonians, Phoenicians, Hebrews, Chinese, Greeks and Romans, as well as Christians all burnt resins like frankincense in their religious ceremonies.

When Moses led the Hebrews out of Egypt, he would have taken his knowledge about oils, herbs and spices to Israel. He was brought up in the palace of the pharaoh, as the adopted son of a princess, and would probably have known about the religious use of oils and perfumes. Several oils, such as hyssop, myrrh, frankincense and spikenard, are referred to in the Old Testament. Olive oil would have been the usual carrier oil at that time in the Middle East. In the Book of Samuel, the prophet anointed Saul as the first king of Israel. Soaking resins or other plant material, such as flowers, stems, leaves or roots, in vegetable oil until it absorbed the resins and essences, could make fragrant oils for religious use. Sometimes the juice of flowers and plants would be squeezed out into the carrier oil.

The Greeks went to Egypt to study medicine and essences and classified and indexed the knowledge of plants. Hippocrates said the way to health was to have an aromatic bath every day. The Romans gave us the word 'perfume', which comes from the Latin per fumum, meaning through the smoke, referring to the burning of incense. Roman soldiers took seeds to the countries they ruled so that herbs, like fennel, parsley, sage, rosemary and thyme, came to Britain. Dioscorides, a Roman who lived in the first century AD, wrote about the uses of five hundred plants in his book, *De Materia Medica*.

In the first millennium, Baghdad became the centre for rose oil from Persia. It is thought that the Arabs were the first to distil ethyl alcohol from fermented sugar, so providing the first alternative method of extracting essential oils using solvents. Damascus also had a perfume industry. In the tenth century, the famous Persian physician, Avicenna, discovered the modern method of distillation. Improving the simple distillation methods of the time, he extended the cooling pipe and coiled it, enabling the vaporized plant molecules and steam to cool more quickly and efficiently. Knowledge about using essential oils and perfumes was brought to Europe by the Crusaders. Monasteries began to grow fragrant plants for their religious and medicinal use. Hildegard of Bingen grew lavender for its oil, and frankincense and pine oils were burned to combat the plague. France became famous for its perfumes.

In the twentieth century, investigation began into the healing properties of essential oils, and the term aromatherapy came into use about 1950. Essential oils are used in beauty therapy, massage, clinical aromatherapy and as a supplement to spiritual healing. All of these therapies work on body, mind and spirit, seeing the body in a holistic way. Used in massage, or in baths or as compresses, the molecules of the essential oils are quickly absorbed through the skin by means of the hair follicles and fine pores. In inhalation, as on a tissue or from a vaporizer, they are absorbed through the olfactory nerve and into the limbic system and then circulated through the nervous system. Often essential oils can get straight to the emotions or places that need healing. Different essences have different properties, on which are based the traditional herbal use. Traditional tales of the way in which gods, goddesses and archetypes are associated with plants and herbs also provide clues to their spiritual use.*

*For much of this information, I have drawn on Shirley Price's AROMATHERAPY WORKBOOK (Thorsons, London, 1993).

Alchemy and Essential Oils

In medieval Europe, alchemy was a philosophy and branch of science that sought to find a way of turning base metal into gold, and to discover the elixir of life, or the philosopher's stone, a universal cure. It is thought today that this was a metaphor for turning the denseness of the physical body into the gold of spiritual enlightenment. Another definition is that it is a synonym for the means of transformation.

Paracelsus, in the sixteenth century, maintained that the main role of alchemy was not to turn base metals into gold, but rather to extract the healing properties of plants. He felt that distillation released the most spiritual essences of the plants, and so aromatherapy can be considered a form of alchemy. As a result of his work, essential oils of cedarwood, cinnamon, frankincense, myrrh, rose, rosemary and sage became well known.

Essential oils, by their very name, are the essences of the plants. In distillation, the spirit of the plant is released and preserved in the essential oil. The more you honour the spirit of the oil, the more it will teach you. We now live in a very technical era, surrounded by the designs of modern technology. Yet we live on a beautiful planet, called by many *Gaia*, or Mother

Earth, for she provides us with all our needs. Even medicines and pharmaceuticals are derived from plants, but the different chemical components are extracted and isolated to provide the relevant medicine. On the other hand, essential oils contain the whole plant essence. It is said that their synergistic affect is more than the sum of the separate components.

If you love gardens, there is refreshment to be found just by walking or sitting among the plants and trees. The scent of the plants and shrubs refresh the senses as the cool breezes or warmth of the sun disperses their scents. All our senses are involved with this experience—touch, taste, scent, seeing and hearing.

The sense of smell is connected to the limbic system, the most primitive part of our brain. It is the basis of our emotions and feelings. The scent of a perfume or plant can instantly recreate our old memories. A client of mine, when I asked her if she would like rose oil in the massage blend, categorically refused. She said she couldn't bear the scent of roses because, when she was ten years old (sixty years previously), her father died. She was forbidden to cry but allowed to throw roses into his grave at the burial. Likewise, the scent of orange blossom (neroli) can instantly transport a woman back in memory to her wedding day, or jasmine to warm summer nights on holiday in tropical countries. Cedarwood or pine oil can bring the memories of celebration during the winter season, with their warming scents.

We can all become alchemists. Through the heaviness and difficulties of the material life darkness can be transformed into light, into the gold of the spirit. By knowing darkness as well as light, we are able to experience transformation. But this can only be experienced with love and joy, through our feelings and emotions, not by the cold analysis of the chemist or by following formulae. So, as Paracelsus said, love is the only thing that opens our hearts. Our daily work needs to be done in a spirit of love and joy, and this attitude is also the one to bring to our work with essential oils.

2. THE CHAKRAS, THE SUBTLE BODY AND OILS IN MEDITATION

Subtle Anatomy and Essential Oils

IN THE traditional spiritual teachings of yoga, it is said that the subtle body, consisting of many layers around the physical body, contains 72,000 *nadis*. A *nadi* is a point in the physical body where energy connects the energy bodies to the physical body. When I was studying Traditional Chinese Medicine on Gabriel Mojay's course, I was fascinated to realize that the *tsubos* (acu-points) of acupuncture, acupressure and shiatsu are also used in yoga. The same places where pressure is placed on the body in a yoga posture are the tsubos where pressure is applied in acupressure and aromatherapy massage. The yoga *asanas* put pressure on the same *tsubos* during the time the posture is held, while using the correct breathing technique, either *mahat pranayama* (full yogic breath) or *ujjayi pranayama* (victorious breath), depending on the posture and tradition being followed.

While it is not possible to have a full discussion of chakras here, there must be an alchemical connection between them and the way in which oils are absorbed from the subtle body, where the chakras are, into the physical body. The seven major chakras are connected to the spine. They connect with the physical body through the endocrine glands, which are the physical counterparts of the chakras. The spine, which is like a tree-trunk, or staff, supports your body. The nerves and circulation system in the physical body and the *nadis* in the subtle body are like the branches and twigs that radiate out and carry energy around them. The firmer and stronger the spine is, the better the posture is, and the better is the circulation of nutrients and subtle life-forces that flow around our bodies.

The ancient yoga texts inform us that there is a subtle energy called *prana* contained in the air we breathe and in the pure food we eat that nourishes our bodies. In the east, it is called *qi* or *chi*. The Hebrews called it *ruarch*. The Greeks referred to it as *pneuma*. All these words carry a subtler message about breath than the English word does. The life-force, then, is carried around the body in the blood circulation and the subtle energy through the *nadis* and chakras. The chakras are 'attached to the spinal column as centres of light rather like bell bell-shaped flowers.' They are 'like receivers…. They seem to absorb, take in, the light; they seem to be where the body breathes in the vital forces' (White Eagle, Spiritual Unfoldment 1).

White Eagle, a twentieth-century spiritual teacher, continues that the centre of the chakra system is the heart chakra, not the head centre of the brain. It is like the sun around which the solar system revolves. 'Then the 'precious jewel within the lotus' quickens and grows. When the oils are inhaled into the respiratory system the subtle essences are taken up into the circulatory system through the heart. When essential oils are applied like perfume* to the pulse points inside the wrists and inner ankles, they connect with some of the tsubos and also the arterial system. When the oil is applied onto the higher chakra points, like the crown of the head, third eye, throat and heart, the spiritual benefits of the oil are absorbed into all the bodies, physical and subtle, or spiritual. (In meditation, use one point only to apply the oils.) Also, during inhalation of the essential oils, they are carried directly into the brain through the limbic system.

*Remember that essential oils should be blended in vegetable oil when used directly on the skin.

Attuning to the Spirit of the Plant Essence

Once when I was in Texas, working with the Native American teachings, my teacher told me to forget what I had been told about the way in which the indigenous peoples had found out the healing and spiritual properties of plants. 'Did you think,' she asked, 'that in those days, the medicine people ate a tiny portion and waited to see what would happen? No, that wasn't how they found out. They sat with the plant and tuned in to it. The plant told them how to use it. We can still do it, if we learn how and practise and if we radiate love and respect to it.'

Dr Edward Bach, who discovered and developed the Bach flower healing essences, also used this method. He developed such sensitivity in body and mind that he would search the fields and hedgerows for flowers that would heal the negative states of mind that he suffered, bringing him back to harmony. Before discovering the particular remedy, he would experience the emotional states that would be healed by the plant.

My teacher got me to sit under trees and ask them to tell me how I could use them. I was amazed at what they said, especially as I did not recognize

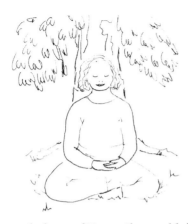

the trees and plants of Texas. She wouldn't tell me what they were until after I had tuned in. So here is the way that you can tune in to plants and their essences. We are so used to reading a reference book or looking up the Internet, we forget we can rely on our own inspiration and intuition. It's a matter of trusting ourselves. Keep a notebook and record your plant attunements or meditations, so you begin to build up a record of what you receive. You will get different ideas whenever you do this. Although this book will give you some ideas to begin with, you can also learn to rely on your own intuition. Share your insights with a group of friends who are also inter-

ested in plants, so a new tradition of plant use can be built up.

In distillation, the spirit of the plant is released and preserved in the essential oil. The more you honour the oil, the more it will teach you. When I use essential oils during my workshops. I choose and dedicate the relevant oil for the purpose, according to the topic of the work, to inspire the participants and release old patterns in order to bring in new wisdom and knowledge.

1.   Choose the plant if you have it, or an essential oil of your choice. Organic or wild plants are best if you can get them. If you use an essential oil, you can use a vaporizer or put one or two drops on a tissue to smell it. You can also use a drop over the third eye (eyebrow centre) or the heart centre at the centre of the chest. Use one drop of the essential oil in a teaspoon of vegetable oil—almond oil or grapeseed oil are easily available at the pharmacist. Jojoba also makes a good base but it will be solid in cold weather. You can blend your mixture in an egg-cup or similar small vessel and cover with cling film, keeping it in the refrigerator for use on another occasion. If the plant is from another country or continent, and no supplies are available here, you can find pictures of the plant to help with your visualization. The

internet is a good source of information and you could print off the picture.

2. Sit in a quiet place where you will not be disturbed. Turn off the phone. If you like meditative music, play some music to create the right atmosphere, especially if you live in a noisy place. Light a candle to represent light. Use a white candle or one that is the colour of the flower or plant.

3. Tune in to your breath. Notice each breath as it comes in and goes out. If your mind wanders, bring it back to the breath.

4. Visualize yourself surrounded by pure white light. The white light reflects silver and gold lights and the colours of the plant or flower. Breathe it in until you feel you are filled by this light and it surrounds you. You find yourself sitting in a sphere of beautiful light. As you continue to focus on your breath and the colours, take them into the centre of your chest, the heart centre, or mind in the heart as White Eagle, the spiritual teacher, calls it.

5. Now bring your attention and intention to the oil or plant. If you know the colour of the flower or plant, visualize the colour. Tune in to it. Think of nothing else and breathe from your heart centre into the plant's energy. You may see the shining form of the plant deva, all light and colour, which will be working with you to use the plant.* Shower the plant with love from your heart, assuring it you will use it only for the highest good. Trust what you are told by it. Be open to any pictures, thoughts, colours, feelings or ideas that come to you.

6. When the meditation is complete, focus your attention back to your breathing. Deepen your breath and start to listen to any sounds around you. Feel your feet on the floor, rub your hands together to create warmth and then cup them over your closed eyes. Massage your brow, cheeks, jaw and chin and then open your eyes and stretch your body. Write down what you experienced. Some of the ideas and meditations I used in this book came to me many years ago, but insights are not lost if written down.

Essential Oil Safety

˙ Never take essential oils internally

˙ Dilute essential oils before using on the skin. As a general rule, useone to two drops of essential oil

*Paracelsus called this the *archeus* (see Mojay, AROMATHERAPY FOR HEALING THE SPIRIT, p. 49). It is the spiritual essence, the life-force of the plant, also called the *qi*.

to one teaspoon (5 mls) of vegetable oil. If your skin is sensitive, use two teaspoons (10 mls) of vegetable oil. Use grapeseed, almond or jojoba, making sure they are of cosmetic quality not cooking oils.

·   Do not use citrus oils on the skin before going out in the sun.

·   Essential oils are not soluble in water, so disperse them vigorously before bathing and use not more than five drops in a bath—less if your skin is sensitive or damaged.

·   In cases of intolerance, if you find essential oils make your skin feel prickly, rub in vegetable oil, like grapeseed or almond, to absorb the essential oil and ease irritation.

·   Use irritating oils in a burner or diffuser only, not on the skin.

·   If you are under medical supervision, always consult a doctor or a qualified clinical aromatherapist before using essential oils.

·   Do not use during pregnancy.

Blending Oils to Vaporize at a Workshop

Choose good quality essential oils, preferably organic. Always look for the Latin (botanical) name to make sure you know what you are buying. If you are not an aromatherapist, your nose will soon get used to inhaling the best quality oils if you visit pharmacies that have good testers, or go to a workshop where you can get used to good quality oils. Remember that the scent of an essential oil may not be quite the same as the plant produces; there is a subtle difference and your nose will soon learn to distinguish it. Also, cheaper and poorer quality oils smell coarser. Good essential oils are more expensive but worthwhile using, especially when chosen for meditation. Begin to learn about blending by putting one drop of essential oil at a time in a small dish. When you get to a pleasant scent, write down your combination. Then you can multiply in the proportion you wish to use. For example, you might decide on a ratio of one drop of eucalyptus to two drops of lavender. Make a times six quantity, and it would last for several sessions when one or two drops are used, so store the oil mix in a small 2.5 or 5ml dropper bottle.

3. SPIRITUAL QUALITIES OF MEDITATION OILS

Angelica root
(Angelica archangelica)

Keynote: *confidence, clarity, spiritual inspiration and connection to angels.*
Affirmation: *I AM surrounded by the loving energy of angels and archangels and their inspiration is always available to me.*

THIS PLANT is well known because the stems are crystallized in sugar and used in cake decoration. It is sometimes called angel's grass.

Angelica is expensive, usually only available in the trade. An aromatherapist may be able to sell you 1 or 2 mls. The plant is called after the archangels 'because of its angelical virtues ... it is a herb of the sun.' (Culpeper) As an herb of the sun, it is associated with Archangel Michael. Like the sword of Archangel Michael, it can help to cut through illusions, helping us to face our shadow self and to develop more spiritually as we become self-aware. It assists in helping us to connect with our spiritual nature.

I burn this oil when connecting with angels and at workshops when needing to attune to higher spiritual vibrations. Invite Archangel Michael and all angels to join you when using it for meditation or if facilitating a workshop. For personal use, it will also help you to connect with your own guardian angel, who is with you from birth. Although many people are able to speak and connect with theirs, others do not know how to connect with them. Use the following meditation to attune to your guardian angel or when you need to contact it for particular advice.

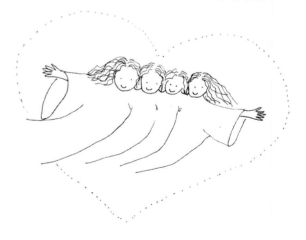

1. Put one or two drops of angelica oil in a vaporizer to scent the air. Centre yourself with gentle breathing. Feel each breath in the nostrils as you breathe in and out. Follow the breath as it enters your chest. Begin to visualize a shining sun above your head. As you breathe in, visualize yourself being filled with light, which floods your whole being. Feel as if every atom and cell is radiating light like millions of tiny suns. Feel yourself rising upwards, as if on wings of light, along a path of light, into the world of light. See this path, as a shaft of light shining in front of you, as you travel up it.

2. You find yourself in a beautiful garden. It is summer and the sun is shining as you walk with bare feet across the grass. The grass feels soft and velvety under your feet. There are beds of flowers of many colours on each side of the path and the warm air is filled with a beautiful scent. You feel filled with peace and tranquillity.

3. In front of you is a magnificent rose arbour with white roses climbing over it. The arbour is built in the shape of a large circle with white trellised panels and an arched entrance, like a temple formed of white roses. Inside are white marble benches. At the centre is a beautiful fountain. The water rises up into the air and rainbow mists form in the spray as the sun catches the water droplets.

4. Sit on one of the benches. Visualize your own personal angel coming to sit beside you and ask for its name. Be open and receptive to any ideas or messages that come to you and don't dismiss them as only imagination. Ask questions or discuss any problems that concern you at this time.

5. Your angel tells you that you don't have just one angel. There is a whole team of angels that works with you in different areas of your life. You are never alone and you have never been alone and they communicate with you in many ways—through dreams, books, ideas, the things people say to you, the songs you hear. Be alert to pictures, ideas or insights.

6. Know that angels of light surround you and the planet earth at this special time. Spiritual strength and inspiration are flowing into us, and the planet, from the spiritual realms that surround us, so that people can make progress in spiritual understanding. Ask, and you will be given all the inspiration you need to help you. This may come in the meditation itself or in some other way at another time.

7. When you feel your meditation is finished, make sure you are centred again (see note 6 on page 14).

Balsam fir
(Abies balsamea)

Keynote: *joy, enlightenment, cleansing.*
Affirmation: *My mind is pure and clear and I am one with all.*

Balsam Fir might be difficult to source, but is inexpensive when you can find it. Fir trees are some of the commonest trees in the world and grow in high altitudes and in the northern hemisphere. The scent of the trees is very fresh and cleansing, particularly on a warm day when the resin is released from the needles and branches. The balsam fir grows in America and Canada, and was used by the Native Americans for medicinal and religious purposes. It is a tonic, bringing cleansing, energy and vitality.

The oil is steam-distilled from the needles and brings the fresh aroma of the Christmas season, the winter solstice, into homes. Fir trees are the trees of choice for Christmas trees. They also bring scents reminiscent of the green forest into the home in the winter, with their uplifting, green and vibrant energy.

The aroma has a stimulating effect on the immune system, bringing mental alertness at a time when the energy is low. For clarity of mind in meditation, drop one or two drops of balsam fir in your aromatic blend.

It also 'opens' the chest, allowing you to take a deeper breath. Deep breathing has an energizing and opening effect on the heart chakra, through its connection with the thymus gland, often known as the higher heart chakra. This connection between the breath, the mind and the heart chakra, enables the meditator to make a spiritual connection with the higher self and yet remain aware and grounded. Balsam fir resonates with the emotion of joy, known in the yoga tradition as bliss (*ananda*), the ultimate goal of our life on planet earth. Joy, bliss, is the goal of the meditator, bringing that sense of at one ment, union with the divine.

There are references to fir in the Bible, such as 'I will put in the desert the cedar and the acacia, the myrtle and the olive. I will set pines in the wasteland, the fir and the cypress together, so that people may see and know, may consider and understand, that the hand of the Lord has done this, that the Holy One of Israel has created it' (Isaiah 41: 19,20).

The Biblical 'Balm of Gilead' is said to be the balsam fir, but a different variety of it. According to *A Modern Herbal* (Mrs Grieve), it is a tree that grows about ten or twelve feet high, rare and difficult to grow. It has been grown in protected gardens in Cairo. It was mentioned by Galen and Dioscorides and exported to Rome at the time of Vespasian. Some stories say the Queen of Sheba gave it to Solomon. Its name of balm derives from balsam in its derivation from the Hebrew, '*bot smin*', 'chief of oils,' or 'sweet smell'.

In my researches into balsam fir, I have found connections between archangels and this oil. (www.4dshift.com/products/html/articles.html) In the Tree of Life model, the position at the centre of the body, the solar plexus chakra and the heart chakra, is known as Tiferet, meaning Beauty or Splendour, and it is associated with Archangel Michael who is full of splendour, like the sun. His name means 'Like Unto God'. This place at the centre of the body is like the sun, around which the other six chakras, like the planets, or archangels (archetypes) revolve (Cortens, WORKING WITH ANGELS). 'But for you who revere my name, the sun of righteousness will rise with healing in its wings.' (Malachi 4:2)

Because of this connection between the opening of the chest and heart chakra, balsam fir, Archangel Michael and his place on the Tree of Life, an ideal meditation is a connection with him. Michael brings you courage and insights into making changes to move on from stagnation in your life.

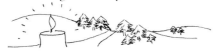

ATTUNEMENT TO ARCHANGEL MICHAEL

1. Sitting in your usual meditation position, begin to centre yourself with your breathing. Follow the breath into your chest and heart centre. Feel yourself bathed in golden sunlight and rising upwards on a ray of light.

2. You find yourself in a beautiful garden among avenues of fine trees. Look around and see a beautiful white building in the distance at the end of one of the vistas. Walk towards it until you are standing in front of it. It is a temple of light, with a finely-carved door and seven steps of clear quartz leading up to it.

3. Climb the steps, feeling the warmth and smoothness of the crystal under your bare feet.

4. When you reach the double doors, there are handles of gold. Turn the handle and open the door. Inside is a beautiful circular hall. The floor is quartz and there are pillars of golden citrine. The roof is open to the light and it pours in, radiating and sparkling onto the crystal. As it does so, the hall reflects all the colours and shades of the spectrum. Vases of roses and lilies stand around the walls and their perfume fills the air.

5. At the centre is a candle, like a pillar, with a still flame burning on it. The candle is level with your

heart centre. There are white benches placed around the walls and you sit on one. The atmosphere is peaceful and you feel refreshed and energized.

6.   Become aware of the presence of Archangel Michael. You might see him as a colour, or as a shining light, a vibration, or as he is usually painted in pictures. However you see him or sense him, you know he is there.

7.   He takes a candle and lights it from the pillar candle, then gives it to you. It is a symbol of light, to show you the way forward in your life. If you are stuck and do not know what to do, you can visualize the way ahead using the light of the candle. Michael asks you what will be the first thing you will do during the coming week to move on and make changes. Tell him any small idea that comes to mind. (Big things start with small steps, or think big and start small.)

8.   It is time to return now. Thanking the Archangel you walk back to the entrance and down the steps, moving back along the ray of light until you find yourself sitting in your room again. Begin to ground yourself by breathing more deeply, feel the solidity of the floor, the ground and start to stretch and open your eyes.

Cedarwood
(Cedrus atlantica)

Keynote: *strength, stability, and endurance.*
Affirmation: *I AM always filled with spiritual strength, the strength to endure through life's greatest challenges.*

Cedarwood oil is inexpensive and it can easily be purchased in a good pharmacy or health store. Cedrus atlantica is the Atlas cedar tree, closely related to the cedar of Lebanon. Cedrus derives from the Arabic word kedron meaning power. The ancient Egyptians used cedarwood as ritual incense and it is often mentioned in the Bible. Cedar of Lebanon was used in the building of Solomon's temple: 'So give orders that cedars of Lebanon will be cut for me' (1 Kings 5:6).

The Tibetans used it as temple incense. The wood is very strong, resisting decay and repelling insects due to the high concentration of essential oil in it. It is good for mental concentration, a useful ability in meditation, when everyday thoughts can distract the mind. I like to think of cedarwood as the pillars of our own temple, the temple of the body, which houses the spirit. Using cedarwood helps to keep us grounded in meditation and yet stills the mind when we feel that our thoughts are scattered.

Spiritually, cedarwood gives immovable strength in times of crisis. It is said to bring the angels of wisdom closer, and will bring the guardian angels closer at times when we need extra strength. (Worwood, THE FRAGRANT HEAVENS, p. 119) This oil, then, can be used any time when you are feeling vulnerable. It is a good oil to keep in the office desk, brief case or handbag. Inhaling a drop of cedarwood oil from a tissue is useful during workplace emergencies or, when travelling, to give strength and confidence in different environments. It can be used as a 'rescue' remedy (not internally). The Bach flower remedy, Rescue Remedy, is an ideal partner to carry with it, and it can be taken by mouth.

When you want to meditate to gain strength and extra insights in a particular situation, burn a drop of cedarwood, or put on a tissue to inhale it, and follow the meditation method on pages 13–14.

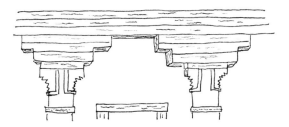

Chamomile
(*Matricaria recutita*, German Chamomile and *Anthemus nobilis*, Roman Chamomile)

Keynotes: *calm, peace, acceptance, serenity.*
Affirmation: *I am at peace.*

This oil is quite expensive, especially German chamomile, but you should be able to find it.

Chamomile is a small herb, of which there are several species. Its fine leaves are feathery and its flowers are rather like daisies. It will grow almost everywhere, but thrives best on sandy soil. When used as a lawn in the garden, its fragrance is released into the air when people walk on it. The two varieties that are used most for distilling essential oil are the German and Roman chamomiles. During vaporization, it fills the air with its delicate aroma. Chamomile tea is a very popular and soothing drink, useful for migraine headaches and gastric problems and as a tonic and analgesic. *Chamomilla* is a homeopathic remedy for toothache and teething in babies. It is also used in perfumes, cosmetics, soaps, shampoos and flavourings.

Chamomile has had over three thousand years of traditional herbal use in the ancient world and the

Mediterranean area. The ancient Egyptians dedicated the herb to the sun, to Ra the sun god. Its sunny associations assist those with sadness, depression and melancholy to feel joy again, in the same way that the sun brings warmth and upliftment after the darkness of a storm. It imparts a sense of peace, calm and serenity to those who have been emotionally distressed.

A variety of chamomile oil was used on the body of Rameses II in 1224 BC as a preparation for burial. Statues of gods, decorated with leaves and flowers, were found in Tutankhamen's tomb. One of these herbs was a variety of chamomile, which was dedicated to the moon due to its soothing and calming abilities, useful when people are angry and irritable and suffering from stress. It is also thought that Christ would have known a Palestinian variety, chamomile anthemus palaestina. Chamomile was dedicated to St Anne, the mother of the Virgin Mary. It represents patience in adversity because of its delicate but hardy nature. It was one of the nine sacred herbs of the Saxons and they called it *maythen*. It is also known as the plant's physician as it promotes health in other plants growing nearby.

The essential oil is blue, due to the presence of azulene, with the German variety being deeper in colour. Blue is associated with the throat chakra, enabling people to express themselves clearly and to work on anger and fear. Because of its association with the sun and the moon as sources of light, it resonates with the body of light. In meditation, it unites us with the Light, helping to soothe and calm agitation, so that meditation becomes easier.

MEDITATION ON PEACE

This meditation is a traditional yoga visualization to bring about serenity. The blue cloudless sky represents the mind without distracting thoughts (clouds). If clouds appear in the sky, just visualize them floating away out of sight.

1. Sprinkle a few drops of chamomile oil into the vaporizer. You can use either or both varieties.
2. Attune to your breathing. If you are tense, begin to notice the gentle calming affect of chamomile as you breathe in its aroma.
3. Visualize the blue sky, still and calm, without any clouds, as on a still summer day. Continue to breathe gently and focus on both your breath, the aroma of the oil and the blue of the sky. If your mind wanders to other things, bring it back.
4. Continue until you feel calm and serene. Then conclude your meditation.

Cinnamon
(*Cinnamomum zeylanicum*)

Keynotes: *joy, warmth.*
Affirmation: *I am filled with joy and confidence.*
Warning: cinnamon should not be used on the skin, as it is an irritant. It is best used in the burner or diffuser.

Cinnamon is well known as a spice in cooking and as burning oil in Christmas spice blends. The aroma of cinnamon, blended with mandarin or orange and balsam fir, cedarwood, or pine essential oils immediately invokes the fun and jollity of the party season, love of family and friends at re-unions and celebrations, and uplifts the spirits during the cold dark days of winter.

It is a very ancient medicinal plant and was used in Egypt in the embalming process. It is frequently mentioned in the Bible, for example, in Exodus 30, where Moses is instructed to make a holy oil that included six-and-a-half pints (four litres) of cinnamon oil. It was to be used in ordination services and was holy because it was dedicated to God. Cinnamon was also known and used in China, where it is mentioned in records dating back to 2700 BC.

Use cinnamon sparingly in the burner or diffuser, as it has a strong aroma that can overpower other oils. It creates a cheerful atmosphere when vaporized with the above oils for parties and functions in the winter.

BASIC BLEND FOR A
SPICY CHRISTMAS BURNING OIL

2 drops of cinnamon essential oil
6 drops of mandarin (or tangerine) oil
4 drops of cedarwood or balsam fir or pine (according to your preference or availability)

Place in a vaporizer with a little water and a tea light under, or in a diffuser or aroma stone.

This blend is ideal for party time during the winter, Christmas and New Year season and brings an atmosphere of warmth and rejuvenation. It lifts the spirits at the darkest time of the year.

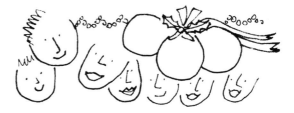

Eucalyptus
(*Eucalyptus globulus*)

Keynotes: *vigour and vitality; cleansing; optimism and openness; adaptability.*
Affirmation: *I am filled with divine energy and strength. My life is in harmony. I do what I love and I love what I do and I do it for the highest good of all.*

The oil is inexpensive and easily obtained at good pharmacies and health food shops. It is contra-indicated during homeopathic treatment. It is best used as an inhalant, as it is quite strong for use on the skin and should first be diluted in a good quality vegetable oil (see pages 13–14).

Eucalyptus is native to Australia, although it is now found everywhere. It is a beautiful tall evergreen tree and there are over seven hundred varieties. Among them are a lemon-scented one, *Eucalyptus citriadora* and a peppermint one, *Eucalyptus dives*. The oil is distilled from the leaves and twigs. The leaves are very tough and leathery, with not much aroma when first attempting to smell them. However, when you rub them hard and bruise them, the scent of the oil is released onto your hands and fills the air. Its oil is well known as an inhalant for chest and lung infections, 'opening' the chest for easier breathing. It is stimulating, soothing and anti-depressant. In the same way as it cleanses and opens the chest, enabling the lungs to take in a deeper breath, psychologically, it allows for openness and more enthusiasm in life. It is a good oil to use when people are feeling restricted in their life choices. It helps people who are timid and want to make changes but can't find the courage to do so. 'It evokes a vital, free-spirited sense of adventure.' (Mojay, Aromatherapy for Healing the Spirit, p. 69)

According to Suzy Chiazzari, in Colour Scents, eucalyptus clears the way for past-life recall and can open the heart to universal love. It enables people to overcome jealousy and envy. Following the ancient doctrine of signatures, the heart shape of the leaves indicates that it is a heart tonic and also cleanses old psychological wounds from the heart, easing depression and emotional heartaches from the past.

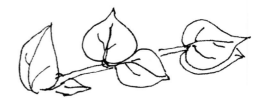

This meditation came to me while sitting under the eucalyptus tree in my garden. It is only a small tree—one in a tub—but I love sitting under it and gazing at the pattern its leaves make against the sky. You might be able to find a eucalyptus tree in your local park and, on a hot day, lie or sit under it, gazing at the pattern of the leaves as they are outlined against the sky. As you idly gaze at this pattern, you might also ask the tree if you may pick some leaves. Crush them in your fingers and hold them to your nose so that you inhale the aroma. Tune in to the tree in the way described previously and be open to any ideas, pictures in your mind, or intuitive thoughts about how the tree will help you. Or sit at home and put a drop or two of the essential oil in a burner.

This meditation is a way of using eucalyptus oil to release any old grievances or grief or hurts from your heart centre (chakra), your emotional self. It will help to heal jealousy or envy and the sort of hurtful thoughts that keep repeating in the mind, try though we might to release the pattern. The symbolism given is that the room you visualize in the meditation is the state of your inner heart. By 'spring-cleaning' it, you cleanse out old hurts.

1. Breathe deeply and take your thoughts into your heart centre. Find yourself standing in front of a door. Take some time to see it clearly. See the door handle and the pattern of the wood. Is it painted or polished? What does the handle of the door look like?

2. Turn the handle and open the door. Go through and find yourself in a beautiful room, but it is neglected and dusty. The room symbolizes the inside of your heart chakra, the energy centre of your heart.

3. Take any cleaning materials you fancy—dusters, polish, a bucket and mop, a vacuum cleaner. Wash and clean the room, opening the windows to let in the fresh air and sweep out the dust and rubbish. Make a bonfire outside to burn the rubbish.

4. When the room is clean, you look around and see a display case with a small beautiful box in it. It is a golden box, decorated with beautiful gemstones, but the gold is tarnished and the gemstones need cleaning, so you clean them and the box.

5. You are curious to see what is in the box. It is locked, but you find a key hanging on a silver chain around your neck. It fits the lock and you open the box. Inside, you see your secret heart centre. This is the place where your secret hopes and dreams are, the ones only you

know about, and also the hurts and grievances you have buried and hidden. It looks neglected and dirty. What material is it made from? Perhaps it is a pink velvet heart, or satin decorated with ribbon or lace, or gemstones. Make it as beautiful as you can and be as sentimental as you like. How can you mend it or clean it? Do this now. Then put this heart centre back into your chest. You don't need the golden box now, because you don't need to lock your heart away, but you can leave it in the room. You have cleaned and polished your heart and feel good. The power of visualization is very strong and, combined with the eucalyptus oil, will certainly help you to find your hidden strength and enthusiasm again. This helps you to connect with your transpersonal self and release old grief and hurt.
6. Conclude your meditation in your usual way.

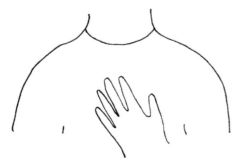

Everlasting (or Immortelle)
(*Helichrysum angustifolium*)

Keynotes: *letting go, releasing, forgiving.*
Affirmation: *I let go and feel safe.*

Everlasting is the name given to the dried flowers that are put in winter arrangements. When the clusters of small yellow flowers are dried they retain their colour, so are everlasting, whence they get their name. It is a traditional European herb that grows in Italy and the Mediterranean. It has powerful healing actions and has similar properties to chamomile. Its oil is one of the most powerful aromatic essences and stimulates the body's own ability to heal itself. It raises the spirits. Because of its relationship to the sunflower, it is often called 'sun gold'.

Both everlasting and chamomile oils regulate the flow of *qi*, or life-force energy. Everlasting also regulates the blood. It is valuable for varicose veins and headaches. It is excellent for severe bruising, as it diverts the flow of blood away from the bruise and disperses it. In the same way, on the emotional level, it can disperse deeply-held energy blockages, like jealousy, anger and resentment, which are symptoms of stagnant *qi*, 'stuck energy'. Everlasting is extremely valuable for those who cannot face deep painful memories, and for those who find it difficult to release their pain by sharing it with a healer, therapist or sympathetic friend. Everlasting assists the sufferer to find inner strength and perseverance in coming to terms with their feelings and memories. It helps to release unresolved feelings and emotions that are dense and buried deep. It can be used, in conjunction with psychotherapy, to releases old defence mechanisms and is comforting in the processing of emotional trauma (www.naturesgift.com).

Everlasting is known as one of the sacred oils, encouraging spirituality and personal growth. The spiritual purpose of everlasting is to make people feel safe. It stimulates intuition and offers encouragement and inspiration for the spiritual journey.

A suitable visualization using everlasting oil is based on the seven-chakra system, those parts of the subtle energy body where these ancient memories are stored. By clearing the chakras of past grief and memories, we can move on. The colours of the chakra flowers given here are from publications of the Bihar School of Yoga, Mungir, India (Swami Satyananda Saraswati, 1993). The visualization is one I experienced spontaneously when teaching about chakras and have often used since. You can do this process lying in the yoga relaxation pose, *savasana*. Be sure to remain awake.

In the yoga tradition referred to, the colours of the chakra flowers are as follows. The names of the chakras are the English ones. The root of the flower is at the spine and the flower opens to the front of the body (except the base chakra and the crown). However, it is said that the positions of the flowers change when you concentrate on them. In meditation, the chakras turn to face up to Heaven, bringing inspiration and spiritual light into the physical body and your everyday life.

CHAKRAS

ROOT (at the base of the spine, the coccyx). Four dark red petals (normally opening towards the earth)
NAVEL (below the navel). Six vermilion petals
SOLAR PLEXUS (above the navel). Ten bright yellow petals
HEART (at the centre of the chest, slightly to the right of the physical heart) twelve blue petals
THROAT—sixteen purple petals
BROW (or third eye)—two silver-grey petals
CROWN (crown of the head, or slightly above)— one thousand bright red petals (opening towards Heaven).

Before you do this, take some time to remember the petals and colours of the chakras and where they are, or read it onto a tape or CD.

1. Put a drop or two of everlasting oil in the vaporizer or on a tissue.

2. Take up the yoga relaxation position, *savasana*, and take some time to relax into it. Attune to your still, quiet and relaxed breath.

3. Take your attention to the base of the spine, the coccyx. Visualize a dark red lotus blossom with four petals. You are looking at it from above because the root is under the spine on the floor. In your mind's eye, examine the petals for any withering or insects in the flower. They are a symbol of a block or disruption of the energy flow in the chakra. (Bees are OK; they represent the gathering of nectar, or *amrit*, a symbol of divine energy.) Visualize the light of the sun shining into the flower. See any withered petals regenerating, insects flying away, until the flower is perfect again.

4. Move up to the position just below the navel. Visualize a vermilion (bright orange) lotus with six petals. As before, look deep into the flower with your mind's eye and check it for withering, bruising, or insects. Visualize the sunlight shining into the flower until it appears perfect.

5. Repeat this process with the solar plexus chakra, above the navel, seeing a bright yellow lotus with ten petals. Repeat with the following chakras:

—the heart with a bright blue lotus with twelve petals

—the throat with sixteen purple petals

—the brow with two silvery-grey petals

Then visualize the crown chakra, and see its thousand (or many) bright red petals opening to the light. The crown chakra is not usually blocked but it may be closed, so open the petals. Visualize the light of the sun shining into it.

6. Return through the chakras, from crown to base, closing all the petals as you go through the visualization*. This closes the chakras. Continue with the relaxation until you feel ready to get up. Roll onto your side and take some time to sit up slowly.

*It is very important to close the chakras before taking up everyday activities, as leaving them open may lead to oversensitivity. A very beneficial therapy to clear old blocked or stagnant energy is Zero Balancing. It can do this without experiencing old, painful memories. See www.zerobalancing.com.

Frankincense
(Boswellia carterii)

Keynote: *tranquillity in contemplation, spiritual freedom.*
Affirmation: *I am refreshed and renewed in the Light.*

Frankincense oil is middle of the range in price and can be found in good health food stores. It is very well known as incense. Its name derives from the French word *franc* meaning 'pure' or 'real' and the Latin *incendo*, meaning 'I burn'. So its name means real incense.

Frankincense is obtained from a tree that grows in the Middle East and Africa. Small incisions are made in the trunk and a milky-white resin, oleoresin, seeps out. The resin hardens into an orange-brown gum. The oil is obtained by steam distillation. It has been used in religious ceremonies for centuries and is probably the oldest known ingredient of incense. The Egyptians used it in the temple incense they used at sunset and also as a cosmetic and fumigant. When burnt, it produced a black powder called kohl, used by Egyptian women as eye shadow and eyeliner.

Jewish ceremonial incense also includes frankincense as one of the four main ingredients. It is the sweet-smelling incense, as the Bible tells us: 'Then the Lord said to Moses, "Take fragrant spices—gum resin, onycha and galbanum—and pure frankincense, all in equal amounts and make a fragrant blend of incense, the work of a perfumer. It is to be salted, pure and sacred.... It shall be most holy to you.... Consider it holy to the Lord."' (Exodus, 30 : 34-35).

Mentioned twenty-two times in the Bible, it was one of the gifts presented by the magi to the infant Jesus Christ, as recognition of his divinity.

Frankincense has an important effect on the mind and spirit, stilling the agitation and worry often experienced in every day life and producing calmness, stillness and tranquillity. It slows and deepens the breath, helping to bring mind and body into the state of unity necessary for meditation. Frankincense holds some of the higher wisdom of the universe and is valuable for connecting with the higher self, the eternal spirit. Use it also if there are seem to be malevolent or negative energies attached to someone, where its high vibration will assist in the removal of these energies. It can also mend a tear or split in the aura, caused by sudden trauma, shock or operations.

Throughout its history, frankincense has been dedicated to many solar deities, such as the Babylonian sun god, Baal, the Egyptian god, Ra, and the

Greek god, Apollo. It enables the focusing of the mind into the spiritual realms. For many years, I have used it as the main ingredient of the oil I blend for workshops and meditation groups. When I add it to the blend, I dedicate it to the Cosmic Christ, the Light. For personal meditations, or when teaching meditation or facilitating groups, I always begin by visualizing Light as a symbol of God/Goddess/Source of All That Is. This light forms a protection during meditation, taking one to the highest possible state of consciousness. In many spiritual traditions Light is regarded as God, or an aspect of the Divine.

'There is a light that shines beyond all things on earth, beyond us all, beyond the heavens, beyond the highest, the very highest heavens. This is the Light that shines in our heart.'* And in St John's Gospel (8 : 12), we read: 'I am the Light of the World'. When Moses saw the burning bush in the desert, he saw it as a sign of God's presence. (Exodus 3).

*Chandogya Upanishad, 3.3.7 (Penguin Classics, 1965)

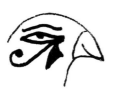 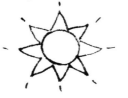

MEDITATION ON LIGHT, USING FRANKINCENSE OIL

1.   Use a few drops of frankincense oil in your vaporizer or on a tissue. Begin to breathe slowly and gently, inhaling the aroma of the oil. Observe the cool air against your nostrils as you breathe in and warm breath as you breathe out.

2.   As you breathe, begin to visualize light shining above your head. You might see it like a spotlight, or a crystal or the blazing sun. Rays of light shine down and around you, as though you are sitting in a pyramid of light. A particularly bright ray shines straight down through your crown chakra, down the *susumna* (the central subtle spinal channel) and into your heart chakra.

3.   Continue to breathe this light and see it filling every atom and cell in your body, even genes in your DNA. As you scan your body and your chakras it seems as if you are radiating light like millions of tiny suns. With each breath, fill yourself with more and more light.

4.   Begin to see a flame in your heart chakra, the light that is hidden within you.

5.   With the next three breaths, as you breathe in, affirm, 'I am in the Light,' then 'The Light is in me', then 'I am Light'.

6. Continue with the threefold breath and affirmations for a short time until you are ready to close your meditation, closing in the usual way.

When you are worried and agitated, use a drop of frankincense on a tissue. After a trying day, put a drop or two in a warm bath before bedtime to help to still the mind and release old memories, because frankincense helps to break from the past. When worried about exams or interviews, put one or two drops of frankincense on a tissue and keep it with you. It will help you to still your thoughts and focus on the questions you have to answer.

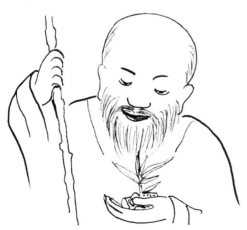

Ginger
(*Zingiber officinalis*)

Keynotes: *initiative, self-esteem, courage and success in achievement.*
Affirmation: *I am happy, confident and successful in all I do.*

Ginger is a tropical perennial herb. Its rhizome is popular in oriental cookery, and ginger tea with lemon is reputed to prevent colds and flu in winter. It is very warming and invigorating and the powdered root is yellow-orange. It was one of the first spices to be brought to Europe from Asia along the Spice Route and was widely used by both the Greeks and the Romans. It is used in traditional Chinese medicine and is reputed to prolong life. Its archetype is the Chinese God of Longevity who wears a yellow robe, the colour of the spice. The essential oil stimulates the appetite and brings warmth to those who particularly feel the winter cold. Its energy inspires people who have plenty of plans and ideas, but never seem to find the energy to do them. In astrology, it is associated with the planet Mars, renowned for its energy, force and vitality. It is valuable when we are physically exhausted and after stress.

Ginger gives courage in times of difficulty and helps the connection to the spiritual realms and the angelic kingdom, especially when we seem to have exhausted all our mental resources. It gives the courage to change direction, to move out of that comfortable rut that nevertheless is a source of boredom, in spite of its comfortable familiarity. The archangelic archetype is Hanael, ruler of Mars and chief lieutenant of Archangel Michael. His name means 'He Who Sees God'. Hanael is red and rules the blood circulation. He is the Archangel of Transformation and Assertiveness. He is a warrior angel, providing energy for successful life processes, reproduction and growth, at all levels, both for mind, body and spirit and all aspects of life. Ginger blends well with balsam fir, Michael's oil, and can be used in the meditation given earlier for Michael. Visualize Hanael with Michael, bringing extra courage when you need to make life-changing plans.

When you have situations where you need to be assertive, use ginger essential oil and meditate with Hanael. Perhaps it is necessary to speak your mind to someone important, or family or friends. You need to state your case clearly and firmly without aggression. The result needs to be for the highest good of all involved, not just for selfish ends.

MEDITATION FOR ASSERTIVENESS WITH GINGER OIL AND ARCHANGEL HANAEL

Put a few drops of ginger oil in your vaporizer and prepare for meditation in your usual way. If you have sensitive skin, ginger can irritate it, so avoid it directly on the skin.

1. Breathing gently and slowly, visualize a path of pure light in front of you. Follow the path and find yourself in a beautiful garden with roses of different shades of Hanael's red colour. Sit down upon a bency put ready for you. Call to Archangel Hanael for help and advice in the situation you wish to resolve.

2. Become aware of a shining figure in beautiful shades of red. The vibrations emanating from him are warm and fill you with courage. Mentally talk to Hanael about the situation you want to change in a way that will be for the highest good of everyone involved.

3. Sit silently, listening for advice and ideas, or observing what pictures or impressions come into your mind. You may just feel optimistic and know things will work out right.

4. When you are ready to leave, thank Hanael and walk out of the garde,n following your path of light, to find yourself back in your body. Be aware of your breath before closing your meditation.

Hyssop
(Hyssopus officinalis)

Keynote: *purification, protection, and fulfilment.*
Affirmation: *I am always in the right place at the right time and always divinely protected.*

Hyssop is strong and should always be diluted in vegetable oil to use on the skin. It may only be found at your local aromatherapist or herbalist. It is a spiritually-purifying herb, mentioned twelve times in the Bible, and is was one of the bitter herbs used to purify Solomon's temple. In the first Passover, it was used to mark the doors with blood, so the angel of death would pass over the houses. Its name comes from its ancient Hebrew name, *ezob*, meaning holy herb. Traditionally, it is known as an herb of protection and is thought to defend both people and buildings from negative energy, hence its use in the purification of Solomon's temple. It is a hot 'herb of fire', ruled by Mars, and stimulates and warms weak, depleted energy, especially good for winter chest infections. It warms and 'opens' the chest and invigorates the nervous system, allowing people to feel more enthusiastic and less melancholy. Its pure, alchemical fire (spirit) action purges negativity from the soul and empowers it, allowing the gold of its spiritual nature to shine.

'Sprinkle me, O Lord, with hyssop, and I shall be purified: wash me and I shall be whiter than snow.'*

SPACE CLEARING WITH HYSSOP OIL.

Hyssop is an ideal oil to use for space clearing, when you want to cleanse a room for a spiritual workshop, and it would work very well with frankincense for this. You can also use hyssop to cleanse the energy of a new house or flat.

1. Thoroughly clean the room or house and if you think there is really dark energy there, you can sprinkle pure sea salt in each corner of the room.
2. Use four or five drops of hyssop oil and vaporize for an hour or until the oil has evaporated.
3. Clean up the salt and open the windows and doors, allowing fresh air and renewed energy into the room. If it's a house, you may want to do each room in turn. You can also play some new age meditation music. Choose spiritual music to encourage angelic and spiritual energy into the room or building.

*From the *Asperges Me*, said during the anointing of the sick (Pre-Vatican 11 Roman Rite, quoted in Worwood, THE FRAGRANT HEAVENS).

Jasmine
(*Jasminum officinalis*)

Keynote: *desire, creativity and harmony.*
Affirmation: *I am in tune with my spirituality. It inspires and guides me.*

Jasmine is very expensive and may be difficult to find. This 'Queen of the Night' is originally from China and Asia and is an ingredient of Chinese jasmine tea. When I was in India, many of the locals wore wreaths of it in their hair or around their necks for parties and celebrations. The little star star-shaped flowers scent the evening air on warm summer nights and they are collected then when their scent is the strongest. Difficulty in extracting the oil is the cause of its high price. It takes large quantities of flowers to extract the oil in a process called enfleurage. Flowers are laid on a thin layer of animal fat, which gradually becomes saturated with the essence and it is then treated with alcohol.

It is a very lengthy process and most jasmine is an absolute, extracted with solvent. The oil may have to be specially ordered for you and, because of the cost, only use one drop in a meditation blend, or by itself for special use. You can also use jasmine oil as a perfume if you like it. Put one or two drops of jasmine absolute in one teaspoon (5mls) of vegetable oil, like almond, peach kernel or apricot and keep in a dropper bottle. You can then put a drop inside the wrists or ankles or on the pulse spots by the neck. These places are by arteries, and the perfume oil is quickly absorbed into the blood stream and carried around the body. If you like its scent, you could wear this when concentrating on creative projects.

Jasmine oil relaxes and calms the nerves. It is an excellent oil to use when you are suffering from nervous anxiety, restlessness and depression and it is said to help develop spirituality. It is reputed to call in angels and help in the connection to joy. Jasmine is associated with fertility and creativity and can be used in honour of Lakshmi, Goddess of wealth, prosperity, abundance and business success. I use it in workshops and when planning them. Lakshmi is the consort of the Hindu God, Vishnu. It is said that Sita, the consort of Rama in the Indian epic, The the *Ramayana*, is an incarnation of Lakshmi. In this tale, Rama, an incarnation of Vishnu, is exiled. His wife, Sita, insists on accompanying him to the forest, where he must stay for fourteen years. She is kidnapped by a wicked demon, Ravana, and taken to the island of Lanka. Rama goes to war, aided by Hanuman, the monkey God, rescues Sita and kills the wicked demon. Then Rama and Sita return to their city, the exile over. Hindus celebrate this event at Diwali, the Festival of Lights, in the autumn. In Asian shops and restaurants, somewhere in the back, you will often see a picture or image of her, with burning incense. The proprietors always know whom to rely on for their success in business! Creativity and success are an important and necessary part in any business.

> 'Giver of boons art thou to all;
> Formidable terror to the wicked;
> Remover of all pain and sorrow,
> Oh, Devi, salutations to thee.'*

Lakshmi, enthroned on a lotus blossom, has four arms. The upper pair each hold a lotus and the lower two give blessings and abundance. She is often depicted with a stream of coins flowing from her hands. She is also known as mother of the world, Lakamata.

For a new business project or venture, use a drop or two of jasmine oil as you meditate for guidance for creativity and inspiration.

*Invocation to Lakshmi, in the *Mahalaksmistotra.*

MEDITATION FOR CREATIVITY AND NEW PROJECTS

1. Place one or two drops of jasmine oil in your vaporizer or diffuser.

2. Begin to breathe and centre yourself. Then visualize yourself being surrounded by Light. Breathe in Light until you are filled and surrounded by Light and you feel that you are radiating Light and all the cells of your body shine like millions of tiny suns.

3. Take your attention into your heart centre and visualize there a beautiful lotus blossom. It is your centre of creativity. You could also visualize Lakshmi as a beautiful woman with four arms, showering you with blessings.

4. Put the idea of your project in the centre of the lotus and wait in the silence for any ideas, pictures, and intuitive thoughts that come to you. Keep visualizing your project in the lotus light until you feel you have finished. Then conclude your meditation.

5. Remember that sometimes the ideas come later. Be open to any dreams or waking thoughts, the things people might say to you. Spiritual guidance is often very subtle and we can miss it. Write down in your notebook what you remember. You may spend a week or a month on getting ideas for a new project, or even longer on major projects.

There is also an abundance mantra for Lakshmi that can be used with the jasmine oil. It is *Om Shrim Maha Lakshmiyei Swaha* (pronunciation: Om Shreem mah ha Laksh-mee-yei swah-ha).

Traditionally, a chant is repeated for forty days, twice a day for twenty minutes at a time—that is, morning and evening—or it can be repeated silently whenever you have the opportunity, as when driving or travelling by train or bus.

Om is the seed sound for the sixth chakra (the brow centre) and is the place where masculine and feminine energy unites. *Shrim* is the seed sound for the principle of abundance, personified by Lakshmi. *Maha* means great, both in quantity and quality, but is in keeping with divine law. For instance, someone might give you gifts but you wouldn't want to be the receiver of stolen goods, so this mantra keeps you within divine right law. *Lakshmi* is the principle of abundance and the personification of wealth. *Swaha* means 'I salute' and manifests energy at the solar plexus chakra, thereby bringing it into everyday manifestation. It also provides a feminine ending to the mantra.

Using this mantra is reputed to process new levels of energy through the chakras. (Ashley-Farrand, HEALING MANTRAS).

Lavender
(*Lavandula officinalis*)

Keynotes: *calm, be at ease with oneself, inner peace*
Affirmation: *I am filled with divine light and peace.*

Lavender is very well known as it grows widely in Europe and the Mediterranean and has been introduced to most parts of the world. It grows well on poor soils and survives drought conditions. Its dried flowers are used in scented bags in drawers and wardrobes. The oil is inexpensive and can be bought almost anywhere, but refer to the Latin name on the label to make sure you are buying genuine oil rather than nature-identical oil, which is synthetic. Lavender lowers blood pressure and slows the heart rate, slows palpitations and is a very useful oil to aid relaxation. It can ease panic attacks. Use one or two drops with a drop of rose otto on a tissue under the pillow after travelling, keeping odd hours, or in jet lag.

Lavender was mentioned by Dioscorides, and Hildegard of Bingen recommended it for maintaining a pure character. Lavender has a reputation *par excellence* for healing. It is an excellent oil to use for people who have a lot of creative potential but lack the courage to follow it up. It is also useful for those who get stuck in the past and can't move on due to old habits. Use it for those occasions when old routines and practices no longer serve their purpose. Lavender is the essential oil 'rescue remedy' and can be kept in the car, handbag or briefcase.

Lavender has the ability to aid spiritual growth by producing a meditative state and it provides psychic protection. It brings about unity between body, mind and spirit. It is good oil in a meditation blend, because it is a psychic cleanser for the meditation space and for those who will be meditating there. It slows down mental chatter and calms stressful breathing so that the breath becomes even and slower, inducing a better state for meditation. For beginners in meditation, or for those who like to practise mindfulness of breath meditation, inhale lavender oil when meditation feels more difficult than usual.

MEDITATION WITH THE BREATH

A simple meditation technique in many traditions is focusing on your breath, so this meditation is based on watching the breath.

1. Prepare your diffuser with lavender oil. Two or three drops will be enough to create the right atmosphere. Sit either in a straight-backed chair or any suitable meditation pose on the floor. Roll your shoulders back and down and lift your chest to enable the breath to flow freely.

2. Close your eyes and begin to breathe gently and silently. Make sure your thoughts are completely centred on your breath and 'watch' each breath as it comes and goes. Keeping your back and chest lifted, but not tense and stiff, watch the breath as it comes into the nostrils, and goes down the throat and chest. Feel the ribs move out followed by the navel as the breath pushes onto the diaphragm. When you feel the natural impulse to breathe out, do so and 'watch' the navel fall, then the ribs and chest come in. Breathe in again when you feel the impulse to do so, but remember not to hold the breath at any time. A similar way to do this is to notice each breath at the tip of the nose as the breath comes in and goes out.

3. Continue to do this with every breath as it comes and goes. If you get out of breath or feel tense, try to relax more. If the mind wanders, just bring it back to the breathing.

4. At first you might only be able to do this breathing meditation for five minutes, but you can gradually build it up until you can do it for twenty minutes. You will find that you will begin to feel calmer and more refreshed. Meditation is best done every day,

but once a week is better than nothing. Another breathing meditation is to count each breath from one to ten and then start again at one. Do this for up to twenty minutes at a time.

5.   Finish your meditation by releasing your attention on the breath, open your eyes and move around the room so you feel grounded again. A drink of water can also help you to feel centred and grounded and prevent the dreamy feeling that might sometimes follow meditation.

'Watching the breath' can also be done with the eyes open if you are tired or stressed. It can be done in traffic jams or in long queues to stay calm. When you breathe in, silently say 'calm', and when you breathe out, say 'relax'. It is also a good practice if you can't sleep. Just lie in bed and watch each breath.

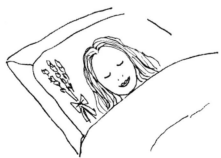

Mandarin
(*Citrus reticulata*)

Keynotes: *gentleness, sweetness of spirit, joy of the inner child.*
Affirmation: *I do wonderful work in a wonderful way and I also find time for rest, fun and play.*

Mandarin, or tangerine, oil is easily available and inexpensive. This variety of the citrus family is native to China and gets its name from the fact that it was traditionally presented to the mandarin as a symbol of good luck, health and wealth. It is a traditional gift at Chinese New Year, when it is given for good luck and wealth in the coming year. In Japan, legends about the fruit of the everlasting fragrant tree are thought to refer to the mandarin tree. The fruit is sweet and tangy and the essential oil is expressed from the peel. It is refreshing and rejuvenating, soothes the nervous system and reduces stress and tension, dispelling depression, intolerance and anxiety. It is relaxing and supportive for those who are workaholics and cannot leave their work behind.

Mandarin is often referred to as 'the little heart of the sun' or 'nature's sunshine', bringing light heartedness to the drudgery of every day tasks. It reawakens a sense of joy and brings a sense of respect to all of life. This is especially true during the dark days of the Winter Solstice, Christmas and New Year, when mandarins are available. You may have found the traditional mandarin orange in the toe of the Christmas stocking you had as a child. The fresh fruitiness of the oil, when blended with cinnamon, cedarwood, pine, or balsam fir, cheers our spirits as we associate the scent with celebrations and parties.

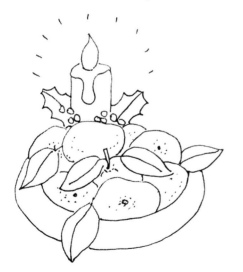

RELAXATION WITH MANDARIN OIL

Mandarin oil is suitable when you need to relax and let go of some of the heaviness and responsibilities of everyday work life. Use it in the following way.

1.   Lie on the floor in the yoga relaxation pose, *savasana*. Play relaxing new new-age music designed specifically for the purpose.

2.   Burn a few drops of mandarin oil. Focus your attention on the breath of relaxation, the easy breath (known in yoga as *sukha pranayama*). In this breath, when you are relaxed, the navel is rising up to the ceiling as you breathe in, falling back towards the floor as you breathe out. Keep all your attention on this breath, noticing each and every breath, navel rising, navel falling.

3.   Remain awake. The benefits of relaxation are different from sleep. Relaxation is a form of meditation, or concentration.

4.   Continue with this for twenty or thirtyminutes.

At times of great stress and tension, daily relaxation can make all the difference to your health and well-being.

May Chang
(Litsea cubeba)

Keynotes: *self-forgiveness, healing, and compassion*
Affirmation: *I forgive myself and I forgive others.*

May Chang is cultivated in China and especially Taiwan. It is not easy to find as an essential oil but is widely used in soap, cosmetics, deodorants, air fresheners and, worldwide, as a source of natural citral. Its lemony fragrance is refreshing, uplifting and stimulating.

I associate the aroma with Kuan Yin, the Chinese Goddess of Mercy and Compassion who embodies the Divine Feminine, an exquisite essence of pure unwavering compassion. In China, Japan, Vietnam and Korea, her temples are often found by rivers or the seashore and in places of natural beauty. She is known as the 'Compassionate One' and is involved in the everyday concerns of men and women. When called upon, she brings divine help to any difficult situation. In the Tibetan Buddhist tradition, she is the feminine aspect of Avalokitesvara, the male Bodhisattva of compassion. Kwan Yin is popular as a Bodhisattva among Buddhists.

TRADITIONAL MEDITATION ON KUAN YIN
This is a traditional meditation, helping to develop our qualities of mercy and compassion. It helps to bring a sense of peace into our own world.
1. Vaporize a drop or two of may chang essential oil or inhale from a tissue.
2. Attune to your breathing. Become still and centred.
3. Imagine it is night. You are sitting overlooking the sea. The night is warm and still and the moon is full. It is reflected in the still water and its light forms a path across the sea. As you gaze at the moon, you feel calm, serene and joyful.
4. The moon grows brighter and brighter. In it you see the form of the goddess Kuan Yin, surrounded by an aura of pure pearly light. You see her clearly as she smiles at you and radiates the qualities of serenity and compassion. As these qualities wash over you and fill you, you realize that compassion towards others heals you also, and that bearing grudges and being judgmental only harms you and no-one else.
5. Repeat her name softly to yourself and observe the feelings of peace and joy that fill you as you do this.
6. Now Kuan Yin begins to leave. The moon is about to set and, as it disappears across the horizon, Kuan Yin also goes. She grows smaller and smaller, until all you see is a small sphere like a pearl.

8. Pearls too are from the sea. Oysters grow beautiful gems around the grit that irritates them. They grow into pearls, the symbol of wisdom. In the same way, the experiences that cause us to be irritable and critical can help us to develop compassion and wisdom, like pearls. Serenity and compassion can grow from our tears and become like pearls of wisdom and beauty.

9. Conclude your meditation but repeat it often to benefit from its qualities of peace, tranquillity and compassion. To gain the benefits of peace and calm, this meditation should be practised regularly.

Once I was given a forgiveness meditation, attributed to Jack Kornfield, a writer about Buddhist mindfulness meditation. This can also be used with Kuan Yin's attributes of compassion and mercy.

I forgive all those people who have hurt or offended me.
I ask forgiveness of (name) (all those people) who I
have offended. I forgive me.

We needn't condone the actions but we can forgive the individual. Self-forgiveness is also very healing and releasing. When we can manage to forgive both ourselves and others, it helps to dissolve some of the darkness and resentment that accumulates around us all.

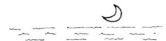

Myrrh
(*Commiphora myrrha*)

Keynote: *tranquillity and peace.*
Affirmation: *I attune to my soul and each day I follow its guidance. I connect to Infinite Wisdom and all is possible.*

Myrrh is a resin collected from a shrub in the Middle East, India and North Africa. The word is derived from an Arabic word, murr, meaning bitter. It belongs to the same botanical family as frankincense. The essential oil is reddish brown and is thick and sticky and is another of the essences reputed to enhance and strengthen spirituality. Myrrh was important to the ancient Egyptians, who used it in unguents and as a funeral incense to burn for the dead. It was said to come from the tears of Horus, the falcon-headed god. The ancient Hebrews drank it with wine to raise their consciousness for religious ceremonies. It was so precious and valued that it was one of the gifts of the Magi to the infant Jesus and it was also used after the crucifixion.

'Nicodemus brought a mixture of myrrh and aloes, about seventy-five pounds..... the two of them wrapped it, with the spices, in strips of linen. This was in accordance with the Jewish burial customs.' (St John 19 : 39)

In addition to its spiritual qualities, myrrh also strengthens the root chakra, helping the sensitive meditator to remain in contact with the earth while making spiritual contact. It calms the nervous system and brings about tranquillity. It stills intrusive mental chatter, enabling deeper meditation. Its use in ancient times as a funeral herb, allowing release of sorrow and grief, is also reflected in its use to help close wounds of rejection and loss. It helps to build the bridge between heaven and earth, bringing the two worlds closer together. As we make the link with our soul, our higher self, we remember who we are and what we came to Earth to do.

MEDITATION WITH MYRRH
Building the bridge to your Higher Self
(your perfected or ideal self)

1. Put a drop or two of myrrh on a tissue or in your diffuser. As the scent of the myrrh begins to fill the air, tune in to your breathing. Be aware of each and every breath. If the mind wanders bring it back.
2. As you breathe, feel yourself surrounded and filled with Light.
3. Gaze into the Light and find yourself in a beautiful garden. It's a large garden, like a park with long, grassy vistas and magnificent trees. There are beautiful flowerbeds and a lake with stately swans. Sit by the lake on a seat you find there.
4. You see coming towards you a beautiful being of Light. It has your face, a beautiful face, the one you might see in your visualizations when you meditate about yourself. It is much more beautiful than the one you might see in the mirror every day. This is the face of your higher self, your perfected self.
5. The being of light comes towards you and its light begins to blend and merge with you. You and your higher self become as one. You are filled with peace and tranquillity as you blend together.
6. Ask any questions that concern you about your earth life. Wait for an answer. If you do not get one now, it may come later, as a dream, waking thought or inspiration.
7. When you are ready, release the visualization and once again become aware of your breathing. Make sure you are grounded before returning to your every day concerns. You have now built the bridge between you and your higher self and should find it easier to connect with your intuition. Repeat the meditation whenever you need inspiration in your life.

Nard, Spikenard
(Nardostachys jatamansi)

Keynote: *devotion, peace, stability, release*
Affirmation: *I am divine Peace.*

This oil is rare and expensive, usually only available from specialist aromatherapy suppliers. When purchasing it, do make sure it is *Nardostachys jatamansi* that you get, as spike lavender (*Lavandula spica*) is also sometimes called spikenard.

Spikenard is native to the Himalayas and is found growing wild in Nepal, Bhutan and Sikkim. It grows at altitudes between three thousand and five thousand metres. The oil is obtained from the rhizome. Spikenard is one of the most ancient and precious of all aromatics, said to be one of the holiest and highest-vibrating substances on the planet and to have many rare and esoteric qualities. It was valued in the Middle East and Mediterranean regions in antiquity. The ancient Egyptians, Hebrews, and Hindus used it for ritual and medical use. It is mentioned in the Song of Songs: 'Your plants are an orchard of pomegranates, with choice fruits, with henna and nard, nard and saffron with every kind of incense' (4: 14).

Spikenard is an oil to connect with the divine feminine, bringing deep inner peace and the understanding that humanity forms a bridge between heaven and earth. It helps in finding that sacred space we all have within, the peace beyond all understanding, found in meditation. It is rejuvenating and excellent to use when tension and anxiety make meditation difficult. It assists the release of old fears and emotional blocks that have been buried deep, bringing freedom of spirit. Spikenard is useful when people are nearing death. Spiritually, it helps to keep in mind the true purpose on earth and to realize that our ordinary, everyday lives are not divorced from it. The oil is useful when searching for the true spiritual path, especially when there is confusion. It is helpful for aid workers and those who are deeply affected by the strife and turmoil seen on news broadcasts or surrounded by crises.

Another use of spikenard is to deepen devotion to a spiritual teacher. Mary Magdalene used it to anoint Christ's feet before the crucifixion and it is seen as evidence of her devotion to him and her understanding of his approaching death.

'Then Mary took about a pint of pure nard, an expensive perfume: she poured it on Jesus' feet and wiped his feet with her hair. And the house was filled with the fragrance of the perfume' (St John 12 : 3).

Recent works about Mary Magdalene refer to nard as a symbol of the highest spiritual essence: 'The oil of spikenard, anoints us all as sons and daughters of the king and queen—royal offspring in our own right, all of one blood, all children of the royal parents—Father–Mother God.' (THE SECRET TEACHINGS OF MARY MAGDALENE, p.85)

The authors of the book also see the use of spikenard as the anointing or 'Christing' of Jesus, as he moved into the final part of his destiny. There is also an ancient tradition that Mary Magdalene and Jesus were married. Nard is said to clean and purify the chakras as part of the ritual of preparation for the sacred marriage, the *Herios Gamos*. In the popular understanding of the seven-chakra system, chakras start at the *muladhara* chakra, at the base of the spine. Another tradition suggests the chakras begin under the feet and rise through the spine through the *susumna nadi*, the subtle spinal channel and ascend above the crown chakra, *sahasrara*. This is suggested as the reason Mary anointed Jesus' feet. Another Eastern tradition is kissing or touching the feet of the guru as a sign of respect. It is certain from the Bible that spikenard (nard) had an important part to play in the story leading up to the crucifixion. It was also one of the spices Mary Magdalene was taking to Jesus' tomb, when she found he had arisen.

In 2004, a worldwide experiment using nard was conducted by James Twyman, through his website, www.emissaryoflight.com. Spiritual changes noted by respondents to the experiment included:

- oneness with the Creator,
- connection to the Higher Self
- connection to new dimensions
- feeling the presence of ascended masters and angels.

A majority of users reported that it brought through the feminine aspects of the Divine.

To use nard oil, you can blend it in a high quality vegetable oil such as sesame or jojoba, in proportion of two drops nard to 10mls jojoba or sesame (not cooking oil). Apply a drop to the nostrils or sniff on a tissue before meditating.

Use the oil before you sleep for enhanced or lucid dreaming; keep some oil with you to use during the day at times of shock or stress; massage your feet or the feet of a friend or partner; place one drop over the heart chakra when meditating on the Divine Presence; use on the third eye (brow chakra) in meditation, or place a drop on the inner ankles or wrists. Spikenard opens the heart and clears away doubts and can always be used to dedicate meditation to Father–Mother God.

Neroli
(*Citrus aurantium*)

Keynotes: *lightness of spirit, regeneration and renewal*
Affirmation: *I am relaxed and refreshed and filled with light, peace and joy.*

Neroli oil is very expensive so should be used very sparingly in the vaporizer. There are cheap adulterated versions available, so check the label for the Latin name to make sure of getting a good quality.

Neroli is extracted from the sweet-scented flowers of the bitter, or Seville, orange tree. Its expense is due to the large number of flowers needed to make it. It has a very sweet and euphoric aroma and a clear golden colour. The flowers are white and very fragrant and the tree produces more than one essential oil. Petitgrain is extracted from the leaves and twigs and bitter orange oil is expressed from the rind of the fruit.

Neroli has feminine qualities and orange blossom is the flower associated with bridal headdresses and carried in bridal bouquets to symbolize purity and innocence. It is named after a princess of Nerola in Italy who used it as a perfume. It was also a constituent of eau-de-Cologne, a popular revitalizing perfume used to revive after fainting fits and relieve headaches in Victorian times.

Neroli's main benefit is as a relaxant and for reviving the nervous system. It helps to relieve the blocked emotions of anger and resentment when they have been ignored and denied. Although known as an aphrodisiac, it also has a very spiritual quality. It unifies the different levels and layers of the subtle bodies, enabling them to come together in unity. The white pure colour of the flowers contains all the colours of the spectrum, absorbed from the light, therefore it resonates with all the chakras, bringing them into unity with the aura after shock and trauma. Valerie Ann Worwood, writing in THE FRAGRANT HEAVENS, notes that its purity touches the angelic realm and it has one of the highest vibrations, as its pure whiteness is filled with light. It liberates the spirit, bringing love and peace.

With its affinity to spirit, to purity and innocence, to the angelic kingdom, and to its white light and golden colour, it immediately suggests Archangel Gabriel. On the Tree of Life model, Gabriel's place is at the base chakra and reproductive area. The sweet perfume of its oil or flowers used in marriage suggests new beginnings and rebirth into a new stage of life. Marriage or partnership or new relationships are a rite of passage, initiating a new phase of responsibility when moving on into adulthood after youth. Neroli is useful to connect in meditation with Archangel Gabriel when you are facing new responsibilities. It creates a different experience from the meetings with Archangels Michael and Hanael, where you need courage, assertiveness and inspiration to make changes. With neroli, the decisions are made, the promises and contracts established. You are feeling a joyful apprehension rather than a timid or fearful one. All you need now is to be able to relax into the enthusiasm for a new phase of life.

The most economical way to use neroli oil is to put one drop on a tissue and inhale the aroma. If you are feeling extravagant, you can use two or three drops in the vaporizer or diffuser.

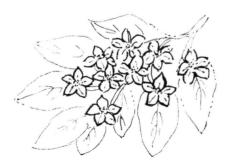

MEDITATION WITH ARCHANGEL GABRIEL FOR NEW BEGINNINGS

If this is for a marriage or permanent partnership, or relationship, your partner could also be involved with this meditation. You could record the instructions and do it together.

1. Sit quietly with the neroli oil on a tissue or in a vaporizer. Allow your breathing to become slow and gentle. Become aware of a feeling of deep relaxation filling you. As your thoughts become still, your breathing becomes deeper.

2. As you relax, you become aware of a shining angel, Archangel Gabriel, before you. You might see it is a being of light, or as conventionally seen in pictures. Its aura is pure and light, scintillating with golden highlights and it is surrounded by rays of light of these colours.

3. The light expands and surrounds you, until you are bathed in pure white and golden light. You feel filled with joy and peace. You are aware that you have come to a turning point in your life and it is right for you. Express any promises you want to make.

4. Gabriel gives you a branch of orange blossom as a symbol of this moment.

When you are ready, conclude your meditation.

Patchouli
(*Pogostemon cablin*)

Keynotes: *grounding, invigorating, stimulating.*
Affirmation: *I am grounded and centred in life.*

The essential oil is inexpensive and should be easy to find. Patchouli is a bushy perennial herb that originates from South-east East Asia. It grows wild in Java and Sumatra at an altitude of nine to eighteen hundred metres. The leaves have a strong aroma and are dried for three days before being distilled. It is used in temples as incense and it grounds and centres the mind in preparation for meditation. Its resonance with the base (root) chakra connects us with the natural beauty of Mother Earth, the planet we live on. Its scent is smoky and earthy. It is also a powerful insect deterrent and, for that reason, dried patchouli leaves were used in the nineteenth century for protecting shawls and fabrics from India and the east that were destined for Europe.

The scent of patchouli is reminiscent of the hippy era of the 1960s and 1970s when the freethinking hippies, who experimented with different aromas of incense, favoured it. They used it to liberate themselves from the old boundaries of the pre-war and post-war era. It was also widely used as a scent and insect deterrent in the eastern-style fashions of the time.

It is a very good essential oil to use for those who are too dreamy, as it helps to ground them. Its aroma also has the reputation of sharpening the mind when, after meditation, we need to continue with everyday things. After we have been inspired by the ideas that come in meditation, it helps us to take the actions that will make them happen. With its strong aroma, some might prefer to blend patchouli with other essential oils. It blends well with may chang, jasmine and sandalwood and also mandarin and lemon.

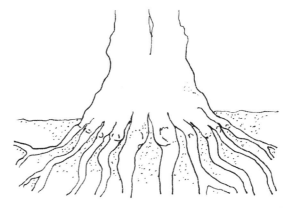

MEDITATION WITH PATCHOULI
for those who feel dreamy and unconnected
with everyday things, and for grounding.

1. Inhale patchouli oil from a tissue or use in your vaporizer or diffuser.
2. Close your eyes and take your attention to the root chakra at the base of the spine, the coccyx (tailbone). This chakra is traditionally associated with the element of earth.
3. Begin to visualize your legs becoming like the trunk of a tree.
4. Breathe out and see your feet growing roots of energy, like filaments of light that stretch down into the earth. With each out breath, see these roots grow right down through the plants, roots and earth, rocks, crystals and gemstones and deep into the centre of the earth, to the energy of its core. Visualize the strength and stability of the planet filling your roots of light.
5. Breathing in, draw that energy and strength back up through the root like filaments and into to the base of the spine.
6. Continue this breathing and visualization technique a few more times.
7. Finally, as you breathe in, bring your attention up to the solar plexus chakra, then the heart chakra to close your meditation.

Peppermint
(Mentha piperita)

Keynote: *attention, concentration, vitality*
Affirmation: *I am refreshed and invigorated. I am able to concentrate and I always know the right thing to do and I make the right decisions.*
Warning: Avoid peppermint oil when using homeopathic treatment and do not store it near homeopathic remedies. Also, refrain from using it in the bath as it irritates delicate mucous membranes.

There are many varieties of mint, and they grow very easily—indeed, they are more difficult to eradicate then to encourage in the garden! Mint likes damp places beside rivers and streams or ponds.

Its name is said to come from the nymph, Minthe, who was courted by Pluto. Persephone, in a jealous rage, changed her into a plant and crushed her into the ground. Pluto turned her into a sweet smelling herb. Nicholas Culpeper, the seventeenth-century herbalist and astrologer, said it was a plant of Venus.

Peppermint oil is inexpensive and easily available. Its scent is fresh, cool and pungent. Mints have been cultivated for centuries and were known in

China and Japan. A type of peppermint was found in Egyptian tombs dating to about three thousand years ago. Hieroglyphs found in the temple at Edfu note it as a ritual perfume and it was one of the ingredients of *kyphi*, the sacred incense. The Greeks and Romans used the herb to scent bathwater and powdered it to use in bedding. According to Pliny, 'the very smell of it alone recovers and refreshes the spirit.'

In St Matthew's Gospel, we read 'You give a tenth of your spices—mint, dill and cumin.' (23 : 23)

Peppermint oil is used in both eastern and western medical and herbal traditions. It is most well known in the treatment of digestive problems and headaches, as an ingredient of toothpaste and mouthwashes, and is very popular in sweets. Refreshing peppermint tea is also easily available in most supermarkets.

The oil is steam-distilled from the fresh leaves. It is very beneficial when studying, or when doing work requiring deep concentration, as it helps concentration and alertness. Menthol, an ingredient of inhalants, is extracted from peppermint. Inhaling or vaporizing the oil assists breathing when suffering from colds, sinusitis or hay fever. It is a useful deterrent on the runs of ants, cockroaches and rodents,

who will avoid areas where it is sprinkled.

Peppermint oil acts on the nervous system, stimulating and awakening both the nerves and the brain, and it is useful when suffering from mental fatigue. It is thus very beneficial when travelling, especially on long journeys and flights. Sprinkle a drop or two on a tissue and keep it in the pocket when on long flights. It is invigorating and energizing and keeps the sinuses free in the stuffy atmosphere of an aeroplane.

It is useful for shock, stress and nervous tension and uplifting for the emotions. Inhaling the oil leaves you feeling fresh and alert.

Emotionally, it gives you confidence to be yourself. It was traditionally classified as a visionary herb and, used in meditation, can bring fresh insights.

Spiritually, it is reputed to stimulate the flow of energy between the heart and the crown chakras and it cleanses and balances the aura. It enhances sensitivity and awareness, so bringing alertness into the spiritual life. It can make the spiritual path clearer so that we gain confidence in following it.

In the yoga tradition, concentration, which is a keynote of peppermint oil, is called *dharana*. It is the first stage of meditation. According to the Indian sage, Patanjali, there are three stages to meditation:

dharana, concentration; *dhyana*, meditation; and *samadhi*, bliss, union with the divine, which is the ultimate goal of yoga.

Often, when new to meditation, people find their mind wandering. Even experienced meditators sometimes find their powers of concentration wavering. One meditator thought he was concentrating very well, and in a state of bliss, until he heard the gong for supper! Use peppermint oil to develop your powers of concentration, but not late at night as it can prevent sleep.

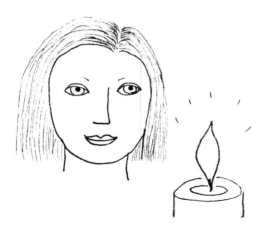

MEDITATION WITH PEPPERMINT OIL

This uses a yoga technique for developing concentration called *trataka*, candle-gazing.

1.   Put a drop or two of peppermint oil on a tissue or in the vaporizer.

2.   Light a candle and place it in front of you so that the candle flame is directly in front of you, two or three feet away.

3.   Sit and gaze at the candle flame without blinking. Continue until you have to blink or tears come into your eyes.

4.   When this happens, close your eyes. You will see the after image of the flame in front of your brow. Continue to gaze at this. If the image disappears, open your eyes and gaze at the flame again, repeating the process as long as you wish.

5.   Then move into a state of meditation.

6.   Visualize a candle flame in your heart chakra and concentrate on it for some minutes. This is also a traditional yoga meditation called *jyhoti*.

7.   Conclude your meditation when you are ready.

Avoid this visualization with the candle if you have epilepsy. Then meditate on the inner vision of a flame with your eyes closed.

Pine
(Pinus sylvestris)

Keynote: *clarity, strength and endurance, self-esteem.*
Affirmation: *I am filled with strength. I am firm and strong.*

This is the Scots pine, which can grow up to forty metres in height. There are over a hundred species of pine trees. The Scots or Norway pine is the commonest variety. The tall trunks of the pine trees were used for the masts of sailing ships. Pine kernels were a favourite food with the ancient Egyptians, who used them in bread, and they are used today in cooking. Pine oil is an excellent tonic for the lungs and 'opens' the chest in cases of chest infections, especially in the winter. This helps to bring about a feeling of self-confidence and a positive attitude to life. Dr Edward Bach recommended the flower essence (not the essential oil) for those who take other people's problems for their own, and to release old guilt and feelings of depression and melancholy. A massage with the oil is also useful for depression and for those who are introverted and withdrawn, encouraging feelings of positivity and self-acceptance.

Pines are enduring trees. Almost all trees have a longer life-span than we do and can see things from a higher perspective. Conifers are among the oldest species on the planet and were the first plants known to produce essential oils. Like cedarwood, pine is used for building and the wood resists fungus and bacteria due to its high resin content. Conifers help in maintaining health, as they boost the immune system. They are reputed to be invaluable at times of transition, such as moving house, changing jobs, marriage, giving birth, and at times of grief and divorce when people need to let go.

As a teenager, I had a very powerful healing experience while being driven through a pine forest. It was the summer of 'A' level exams and I had a terrible attack of catarrh and sinusitis. I could hardly breathe, my head ached and nothing seemed to relieve it. We went on a visit to Edinburgh, driving up through the pine forests of Cumbria and southern Scotland. The day was hot and sunny and we had the car windows open. The scent of the pine trees was like perfume and by the time we arrived, my stuffy nose and headache were completely cured. This was just before I left home to go to college, a time when I needed a secure sense of direction, on the verge of adulthood. Pine certainly gave it to me. Pine trees also have the reputation of healing the energy field.

Pine oil is very good for massaging the lower back when it feels achy and weak. In yoga postures, the sitting posture is called *dandasana*, the staff, or stick pose. The staff referred to is the spine, which keeps us strong and erect, just as a pilgrim's or shaman's staff helps them. Sit on the floor, with your legs straight out in front of you and rest your hands beside you, palms to the floor and your spine lifted and straight. A pine oil massage strengthens the spine, your own staff.

In parts of Poland and the Czech Republic, pine resin was burnt between Christmas and New Year to deter evil spirits and other negative influences. In some parts of Europe, pine trees are planted around cemeteries. There are Japanese myths about the fungus of immortality, which grows under holy trees, thought to be pine trees. In China, dragons, which are thought to bring good luck, are associated with pine trees. It is said that pine trees change into dragons.

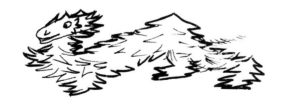

MEDITATION AMONG THE PINES

1.   If you know a safe place amongst pine trees where you could meditate, sitting with your back against a pine tree, it would be ideal. It is, in any case, very strengthening to stand with your back against a tree. I have a favourite cedar tree in my local park and I like to lean against its trunk. Otherwise prepare your oil as before.

2.   Centre yourself with your breathing in the usual way, becoming aware of the invigorating aroma of the pine essence.

3.   Visualize yourself sitting in a pine forest. Inhale the aroma of the pine trees. Imagine yourself sitting with your back to a strong pine trunk. Feel the firmness of the bark against your back. Feel the strength of the tree filling your own 'staff' (spine) and invigorating it with its energy.

4.   Look around you and see that you are in a clearing in the pine forest. The trunks of the majestic trees are like the columns of a natural cathedral.

5.   In the centre of the clearing you become aware of a shaft of bright light. As you become accustomed to it, you see the form of an angel, or deva, of the pine forest. It envelops you with strengthening healing energy. You know that its spiritual essence of strength

and confidence is also present in the oil when you use it.

6. The angel surrounds and fills you with strength and healing and you in turn radiate your love and gratitude to the angel and for the gifts of the trees.

7. When you feel your meditation is complete, thank the angel and the trees for their gifts of strength and endurance.

8. Conclude your meditation.

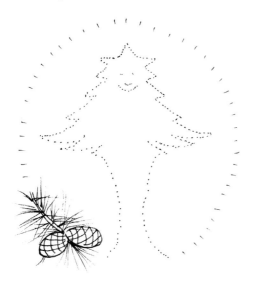

Rose
(Rosa Damascena)

Keynote: *love and devotion, inner vision, self acceptance.*

Affirmation: *May the jewel in the rose of my heart burn brightly, bringing about spiritual illumination.*

The damask rose produces the best quality essence, rose otto. As this oil is costly, use the solvent-extracted absolute in the vaporizer. Two other roses are also used for perfume, *Rosa centifolia*, the cabbage rose and *Rosa gallica*, the French rose.

The rose is, perhaps, the most popular flower of all. Entire books are written about the rose, from its cultivation, myths and tradition, to perfumery and essences. Sappho, the Greek poetess, called the rose 'queen of flowers' over two thousand years ago. The history of the rose can be traced back for hundreds of years. Fossil records show roses already in existence forty million years ago. The oldest image of roses is found on the wall of the Palace of Knossos, excavated in Crete. A Hittite coin also shows a rose stamped on it and is believed to date from 2,000 BCE. In 1888, Sir Flinders Petrie, the British archaeologist, discovered a wreath of five-petalled flowers in an Egyptian tomb. Although shrivelled in the dry desert air, they had kept their colour. When placed in warm water, they seemed to revive. 'The buds swelled and the pink petals spread, unfolding to reveal the knot of golden threads at the centre, just as they must have been on the morning of the funeral.' (Lawless, Rose Oil, p. x) It was identified as *Rosa sancta*, the Holy Rose of Abyssinia (Ethiopia).

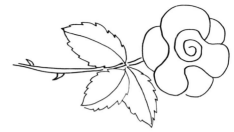

The rose is one of the flowers sacred to the Egyptian Goddess, Isis. It is reported that rose petals were strewn eight inches deep on the ground when Cleopatra first met Mark Antony. Greeks dedicated the rose to Aphrodite, Goddess of love and beauty. The Romans linked the rose with Venus, Goddess of Love. Signs of an ancient rose cult have also been found in India and Syria. The name, Syria, derives from 'suri', meaning land of roses. The rose is a powerful symbol and is used all over the world to suggest love, but also inspired the name of 'the Wars of the Roses' in medieval England. In medieval times, also, roses were sacred to Mother Mary, the mother of Jesus Christ. A well-known carol from this period is often sung during the Christmas season.

'There is no rose of such virtue
As is the rose that bare Jesu.'

The rosary, the beads on which prayers are said to Mary, gets its name from roses. They were originally made from a hundred and sixty-five dried and carefully-rolled rose petals. The wild rose is still the royal flower of England and the British King or Queen is anointed at the coronation ceremony with a holy oil containing rose essence. The recipe dates back to the twelfth century. A single red rose is given as a token of love and bouquets of red roses fill the florist's and supermarkets on St Valentine's Day.

Culpeper considered the rose to be a cephalic herb—that is, it is uplifting to the mind in depression. It is also helpful for insomnia, as it quietens the mind. In traditional aromatherapy, the rose (*Rosa damascena*, rose otto) is used as a heart tonic. It calms and supports the heart and restores a sense of well-being. 'The damask rose is the Holy Rose, a symbol of God's love to the world.' (Mojay, Aromatherapy for Healing the Spirit, p. 113). When Bernadette had her vision of Mary at Lourdes, she was surrounded by roses.

As well as being associated with the physical heart in the western mystery tradition, the rose is taken as a symbol of the heart chakra, the energy centre associated with the physical heart and the thymus gland. In the yogic tradition, the lotus blossom has the same significance but, from ancient times, the heart chakra is seen as the centre of the spirit.

'In the centre of the castle of Brahman, our own body, there is a small shrine in the form of a (lotus) flower.... The little space within the heart is as great as this vast universe ... for the whole universe is in him and He dwells within our heart.' (CHANDOGYA UPANISHAD, Penguin Books, 1977)

In 'The Song of Songs,' the bride of the songs speaks: 'I am a rose of Sharon' (2 : .1)

In a recent book (THE SECRET TEACHINGS OF MARY MAGDALENE), Claire Nahmad and Margaret Bailey take the Rose of Sharon to be Mary Magdalene or even Isis herself. The rose symbolizes the spirit. *Shar-on* is considered to be an Orbit of Light, 'an inner world of the spiritual realms associated with advanced enlightenment.' The lily upon the surface of the water is taken as a symbol of spirit and the rose is its innermost centre, the jewel at the heart of the lotus.

The spiritual teacher, White Eagle, speaking through Grace Cooke, spoke often of the rose. He reminded his students of the Rosicrucian Brotherhood, whose greeting was 'may the rose bloom upon your cross'. This meant that through constant striving towards the Light, the darkness of materiality, the cross, (astrological symbol of planet Earth) would be transmuted into the fragrant rose of the spiritual life (*Stella Polaris*, August–September 1962, White Eagle Publishing Trust.) He referred to Christ as the Master of the Rose.

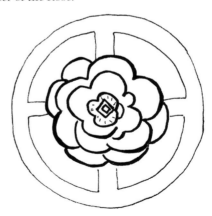

MEDITATION ON THE ROSE

1.　Sit for meditation as described (pp. 13–14), using rose oil.

2.　Visualize a brilliant light like the sun or a radiant star shining above you. Breathe in its light and feel it shining down through your crown centre (chakra) into your chest and heart chakra.

3.　Continue to breathe in this light and see it shining on to a beautiful rosebud in the centre of your chest, the heart chakra. Observe the rose and its colour.

4.　As the light continues to shine onto the rose, see the petals begin to open. The petals open wide. Deep in the heart, your heart, of the rose, you see a small drop of dew. The light pours down onto the drop of dew and it becomes brilliant like a diamond.

5.　The rose becomes a full-blown rose with a brilliant diamond, the jewel of enlightenment, deep in its heart. This diamond, the jewel of the Christ, of enlightenment, of Brahman, or the Great Spirit, is always there, waiting to be discovered and revealed. Then we truly know ourselves.

6.　When you are ready to close your meditation, visualize the petals of the rose closing again to protect the jewel.

7.　Bring your attention back to the breath, then open your eyes when ready.

Rosemary
(*Rosemarinus officinalis*)

Keynotes: *self-knowledge, dedication, and destiny. It is an herb of remembrance.*
Affirmation: *I remember who I am, where I am from, why I am here, where I am going.*
Warning: Rosemary oil should not be used in cases of epilepsy or during pregnancy. However, in such cases, it is safe to use the herb in cooking.

Many of us probably remember the well-known keynote mention of rosemary in the words, 'There's rosemary, that's for remembrance', which are from Ophelia's speech in *Hamlet*. Culpeper recommended it to help a weak memory and to quicken the senses. It is associated with the sun, which brings vitality.

Rosemary oil is easily obtainable and is inexpensive. Rosemary is a very popular culinary herb. It is an evergreen perennial shrub, with leathery green spiky leaves and pale blue flowers in springtime. Its name, rosemary, is derived from the Latin *Ros marinus*, meaning rose of the sea. Sprigs of it can be soaked in vinegars and olive oil to impart its properties for cooking and a herbal massage oil can be made from it by infusing the sprigs in a vegetable oil.

The ancient Egyptians burnt sprigs of rosemary as ritual incense and placed them in the tombs of the pharaohs to help them remember their former life. The plant was also sacred to the Greeks and Romans. The Greeks dedicated it to Apollo, the sun god, and the god too of medicine, music, poetry and prophecy. It symbolized loyalty, death and remembrance, as well as scholarly learning. People wore garlands of rosemary at weddings and important occasions to symbolize trust and faithfulness. This custom continued in Europe, as sprigs of gilded rosemary were presented to guests to symbolize love and friendship. It was burnt as incense at funerals to respect and honour the deceased. Rosemary has been associated with good luck for centuries and is also known as an herb of protection. In medieval times, it was used to protect against the plague and also as a tonic to improve health. Rosemary also assists the work of healing angels and it protects psychically. Use one drop of the oil on a tissue, or in the water you wash with in the morning if you are travelling on public transport, working in a busy office or dealing with the public. It is also a stimulant, waking you up ready for the day.

Used in meditation, it brings confidence and self-worth. It is an excellent oil to use for those who dismiss their meditations as 'only imagination' and lack confidence in their inner guidance. For such people, burning or using the oil on a tissue will help to make the spiritual connection needed during meditation. It will help them to become more confident in using and trusting the guidance that comes to them. The oil helps us to remember who we really are, that we are spiritual beings having a human experience (see the affirmation above). It has an affinity with the brow chakra, known as the third eye, *ajna chakra* in the yogic system. This is the chakra particularly associated with the intuition and inner vision. Modern education does not encourage the use of the imagination. When I am teaching workshops and meditation, I often ask how many people were reprimanded for daydreaming at school when they were young. There is usually a one-hundred-percent response. Were you told to stop daydreaming and to pay attention to the lesson in progress? That is one way to lose the connection with your spiritual self, which communicates through the imagination and intuitive guidance.

'Imagination is truly the doorway to your creative powers. It is primarily a spiritual thing and opens up a higher world.' (White Eagle)

White Eagle has a lot to say about imagination.

He reminds us that when we see pictures in our minds and imagine them clearly, we are developing spiritual clairvoyance. We need to use the act of will to go into the world of imagination and eventually we will realize we are visiting the world of spirit. He tells us that, when we think 'it is only my imagination', it is really the lower mind speaking and it is our enemy. So using rosemary oil helps to remind us that we do come from the world of spirit, and we will return there, but also we can go there now in meditation. Rosemary also helps with developing clarity in using the will in creative visualization.

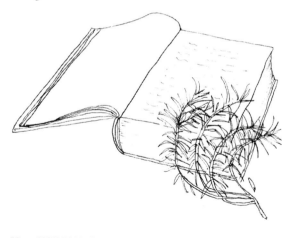

VISUALIZATION TO CONNECT WITH YOUR LIFE PURPOSE

1. Use the essential oil as before and breathe slowly and smoothly. Think of nothing but your breath. Witness each breath as it comes and goes.
2. Visualize light surrounding you and filling you until you feel every atom and cell of your whole being resonating with light.
3. See in front of you a shining being of light, your guardian (or personal) angel. Imagine it clearly. What colours is it wearing or what coloured light is it? How do you feel? (peaceful, happy, confident, loving?) What other positive feelings might you feel? This is the keynote of your personal angel.
4. The angel takes you through the light until you see in front of you a magnificent building. It is a library of records. What does it look like? Is it like a university, a city library, a civic building? Create it in your mind. Decide what the architecture is like, the doors, windows, steps to the entrance. In it you will find your Book of Life, which records all you agreed to do before you returned to this earth life.
5. Go into the magnificent building with your angel. Inside there is a large reception area with corridors leading from it. Follow the angel along one of

the corridors. Observe the furnishings and decorations. There are doors along the corridor. What do they look like? You come to a door with your own name on it. This is where the records of your life are held.

6. Go into the room and inside you see a large table. On it is a book, your Book of Life. There is a curator or wise man–woman there, your spirit guide. Your guide and guardian angel help you with your life mission. When you ask for help, they will always help you. The book is open, at a page that tells you what you decided to do in this life before you were born. The guide and angel helped you to choose your parents and the conditions you would need in life. You even decided your name.

7. Read the page that is open before you. If you feel you need help with your life, ask for guidance. If you already know what your life work is, ask for help to complete it successfully.

8. Thank your guide and angel and leave the room, walking along the corridor and back to the reception area and out of the building. You can return any time you need more inspiration.

You find yourself back in your body. Breathe more deeply and make sure you are grounded again. Affirm, 'I remember my life's purpose'.

Sandalwood
(*Santalum album*)

Keynote: *stillness, serenity, unity.*
Affirmation: *I am in tune with divine wisdom.*

Sandalwood is becoming more rare and expensive, owing to over-felling of the trees. Beware of adulterated oils and substitutes from other areas. You need to check the correct botanical name when buying the oil and buy only from a reputable aromatherapy supplier.

Sandalwood is a parasitic evergreen tree, which grows to a height of about nine metres. The best oil is extracted from the heartwood by steam distillation and is pale yellow in colour.

The tree is found in Southern Asia and the best medicinal quality is found in Mysore. The wood is carved into furniture, temples, statues and images, *mala* (meditation) beads and is burnt as incense in Buddhist and Hindu temples. It is used to anoint and embalm the dead and to carry the soul onto its journey into the next life. Yogis use it to encourage the state of meditation and enhance devotion to the divine and it is widely used in ceremonies.

It balances the energy between the base and crown chakras. The oldest record of sandalwood is found in the Vedic scripture, the *Nurukta* (fifth century CE), and it is mentioned as one of the most valuable essences of Indian spiritual use.

Its aroma is said to reach out into the universe finding spiritual wisdom and inspiration. At the emotional level, it encourages warmth, sensitivity, harmony, peace, wisdom and unity within oneself and with the divine. The effect of its oil is soothing and very relaxing, while for those who lack self-esteem, sandalwood is a good oil to have. This lack often stems from childhood, when children can feel as if they are no good and can do nothing right.

I associate sandalwood with Saraswati, goddess of wisdom and learning. She is usually depicted sitting on a lotus pedestal, with four arms. She plays a *veena*, a one-stringed lute, with two of her hands. In the upper right hand she holds a rosary, while in the upper left hand she holds a book. Her vehicle is a swan, a symbol of grace and her emblem is a six-pointed star, the yogic symbol of the heart chakra.

In the western traditions, Sophia is the goddess of wisdom. Sophia is her Greek name. In Hebrew it is Hokhmah, and she is seen as the feminine aspect of God. Her symbol is the dove, representing the Holy Spirit. She is seen crowned by stars. In the Biblical traditions, she is often associated with Solomon, the wise King of Israel. In the Book of Kings, we are told that God gave wisdom to Solomon and, in the Song of Songs, it speaks of Solomon's marriage to Holy Sophia. She is particularly worshipped in the Eastern and Russian Orthodox traditions and venerated in the Gnostic tradition. She is often linked to Mother Mary and Mary Magdalene and is also depicted as the Egyptian Goddess, Isis.

So sandalwood oil has a strong association with feminine divine wisdom, and can be used when you especially want to attune to wisdom for a particular project or idea. However, as sandalwood is also a sedative, to prevent sleep only use one or two drops. The spiritual teacher, White Eagle, tells us that the colour of spiritual wisdom is yellow, the colour also of sandalwood oil. He also says that true wisdom cannot be learned, it is innate. Reading all the books in the world will not make us wise but, when we meditate, we can contact divine wisdom.

MEDITATION ON SPIRITUAL WISDOM WITH SANDALWOOD OIL

1. Use the oil as before. If you can find a yellow or orange rose, place it in front of you. The rose is the symbol of the heart, the place of wisdom. White Eagle calls it the mind in the heart.

2. Gaze at the rose and begin to breathe slowly and gently. The breath in meditation should always be smooth.

3. Close your eyes and continue to visualize the rose. Then visualize the rose being in your heart chakra and breathe in and out of the rose.

4. Begin to feel that the rose is growing bigger and bigger until you are inside the rose. Inhale the scent of the rose and see the petals turning into pillars of a beautiful temple of wisdom. Look around you and become aware of beautiful golden light surrounding you. You may become aware of some of the symbols of wisdom mentioned earlier.

5. Continue to breathe in this pure golden light, the light of pure spiritual wisdom. If there are any issues that you would like some enlightenment about, concentrate on them and wait for pictures, images, ideas, that come into your mind. Don't dismiss them as 'only imagination.'

6. You might become aware of a shining goddess figure who speaks to you.

7. Continue to visualize and breathe gently into your heart chakra until you feel it's time to conclude.

8. Bring your attention back to the breath, release the imagery, and when you are ready, open your eyes.

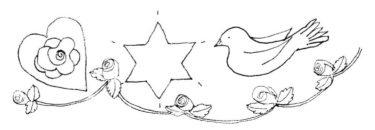

4. CONCLUSION

MANY MORE essential oils could be used for meditation. The ones mentioned are those that I have used for many years and with which I have experienced the meditations given. Once you become interested in using essential oils to meditate with, you will find that you become more and more enthusiastic and inspired. Use the oils when you meditate, follow the processes given and discover more and more information from the plant world. Keep a notebook and build up a *materia aromatica* of information, for your own use if for no-one else. The alchemy of essential oils begins at home, with the plants we know and use often.

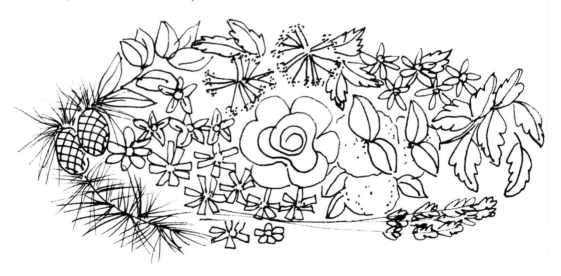

Appendix

KEYS Meditation Blend

I have formulated a blend that we use for meditation at our workshops and meditation groups. It contains eleven of the essential oils mentioned in the book.

For more information, please contact us through our website www.keystolight.co.uk or phone +44 (0)20 8560 7201. We also sell CDs of music for meditation including singing bowls, essential oils and books, and we teach yoga and workshops of a spiritual nature. Contact us through the website or phone.

Bibliography

Ashley-Farrand, Thomas: HEALING MANTRAS, with CD (Gateway, 2000)

Chiazzari, Suzy: COLOUR SCENTS (The C.W. Daniel Company, 1998)

Cooke, Grace: MEDITATION (third edition, White Eagle Publishing Trust, 1999)

Cooke, Grace: THE JEWEL IN THE LOTUS (White Eagle Publishing Trust, 1973)

Cortens, Theolyn: WORKING WITH YOUR GUARDIAN ANGELS (Piatkus, 2005)

Cortens, Theolyn: WORKING WITH ANGELS (Caer Sidi Publications, 1996)

Culpeper, Nicholas: CULPEPER'S COLOUR HERBAL (Foulsham, 1996)

Davies, Patricia: SUBTLE AROMATHERAPY (The C.W. Daniel Company, 1991)

Hayward, Ylana: A WAY TO HAPPINESS (White Eagle Publishing Trust, 1995)

Howard, Judy: THE BACH FLOWER REMEDIES STEP BY STEP (The C.W. Daniel Company, 1990)

Lawless, Julia: ROSE OIL (Thorsons, 1995)

Lawless, Julia: THE ILLUSTRATED ENCYCLOPEDIA OF ESSENTIAL OILS (Element, 1996)

Majupuria, T.C., and Rohit Kumar (Majupuria) GODS AND GODDESSES (Smt. M.D. Gupta, India, 2000)

Mojay, Gabriel; AROMATHERAPY FOR HEALING THE SPIRIT (Gaia Books, 1996)

Nahmad, Claire and Bailey, Margaret: THE SECRET TEACHINGS OF MARY MAGDALENE (Watkins, 2006)

Prabhavananda, Swami, and Manchester, Frederick: THE UPANISHADS, BREATH OF THE ETERNAL (Mentor, 1980)

Price, Shirley: AROMATHERAPY WORKBOOK (Thorsons, 1993)

Satyananda, Swami: YOGA NIDRA (Bihar School of Yoga, Bhargava Bhushan Press, Varanasi, 1993)

The Bible: New International Version, Hodder & Stoughton, 1996

White Eagle, SPIRITUAL UNFOLDMENT 1 (White Eagle Publishing Trust, third edition, 2000)

Wildwood, Chrissie: AROMA REMEDIES (Collins and Brown, 2000)

Wildwood, Chrissie: CREATE YOUR OWN PERFUMES USING ESSENTIAL OILS (Piatkus, 1994)

Worwood, Valerie Ann: THE FRAGRANT HEAVENS (Bantam Books, 1999).

UK Suppliers of Essential Oils and Equipment

Alan Howell, Shechina, 21, Chatsworth Crescent, Hounslow, Middlesex, TW3 2PE
Tel. & fax +44 (0)845 458 5757
www.shechina.co.uk
Natural by Nature Oils
www.naturalbynature.co.uk
Essentially Oils
www.essentiallyoils.com

Materia Aromatica, essential oils from organic and wild-crafted plants, London House, 42c Upper Richmond Road West, London SW14 8DD.
Order line: 020 8392 9868
www.materiaaromaatica.com

Outside the UK, try www.naturesgift.com (Nature's Gift Aromatherapy in Tennessee, USA, or key 'essential oils' into an internet search engine.

Useful Websites

KEYS, Kathleen and Roy Pepper:
www.keystolight.co.uk
Theolyn Cortens:
www.soulschool.co.uk
The Zero Balancing Association:
www.zerobalancing.com
The Institute of Traditional Herbal Medicine and Aromatherapy:
www.aromatherapy-studies.com
James Twyman's site (see p. 44):
www.emissaryoflight.com
The White Eagle Lodge:
www.whiteeagle.org
Polair Publishing
www.polairpublishing.co.uk